BARBARA WINTROUB

WITH
DANIEL WILSON

FIGHTING GRAVITY

A GUIDE TO EXTENDING THE WARRANTY ON YOUR BODY

T0171426

Balboa Press books may be ordered through booksellers or by contacting:

Balboa Press

BALBOA.
PRESS
A DIVISION OF HAY HOUSE

A Division of Hay House
1663 Liberty Drive
Bloomington, IN 47403
www.balboapress.com
1-(877) 407-4847

Barbara Wintroub, Active Aging Expert
www.retrofitpilates.com
bwintroub@retrofitpilates.com

ISBN: 978-1-4525-3653-8 (e)
ISBN: 978-1-4525-3652-1 (sc)

Library of Congress Control Number: 2011911156

Printed in the United States of America

Balboa Press rev. date: 7/12/2011

I WANT TO THANK MY PARENTS WHO TAUGHT ME TO STAND UP STRAIGHT MAKING IT EASIER TO DO AS I GET OLDER.

THANK YOU TO ALL THOSE FRIENDS AND CLIENTS WHO HAVE CONTRIBUTED TO THE KNOWLEDGE I HAVE TODAY ON AGING.

THANK YOU TO DANIEL WILSON, WRITER FOR BALANCED BODY, INC., WHO TOOK MY WORDS AND MADE THEM INTO A BOOK.

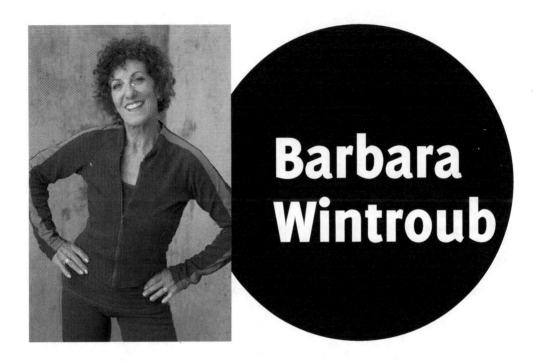

Barbara Wintroub graduated California State University, Northridge with a degree in Kinesiology. She has a lifetime State of California Teaching Credential, is currently a Faculty Member with UCLA Extension-Personal Training Dept., Balanced Body University, American Council on Exercise (ACE) and has taught over 400 Physical Therapists how to incorporate Pilates into their PT program.

Certifications:
First Tier Member of the Pilates Method Alliance (PMA), Gyrotonic Expansion System, American Bone Health, Degreed Personal Fitness Trainer, Medical Exercise Specialist with American Academy of Health, Fitness and Rehabilitation Professionals (AAHFRP), Pilates for Golf and Nordic Walking.

As a member of the BABY BOOMER GENERATION, Barbara is considered an "Active Aging Expert." She has recently been selected to be a member of the Visioning Board for the International Council on Active Aging (ICAA), coming up with breakthrough ideas to motivate people to become fit. Barbara now lives in Palm Desert, California where she continues to present new material on Osteoporosis and Alzheimer's disease exercise programs and teaches Truckers how to exercise behind the steering wheel.

Barbara is a nationally ranked tennis and pickleball player, Ironman triathlete and she is one of the first 40 women worldwide to have run a marathon on all 7 continents.

"SOMETIMES THE BEST WAY TO FIGURE OUT WHO YOU ARE IS TO GET TO THAT PLACE WHERE YOU DON'T HAVE TO BE ANYTHING ELSE."

— UNKNOWN

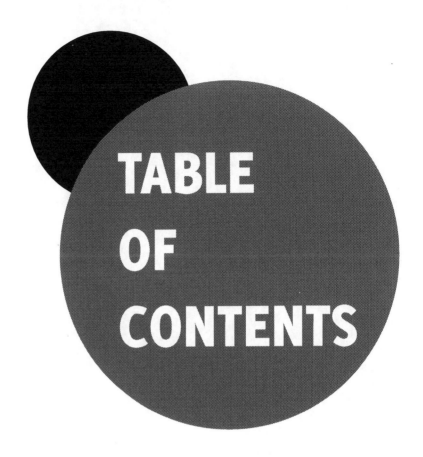

TABLE OF CONTENTS

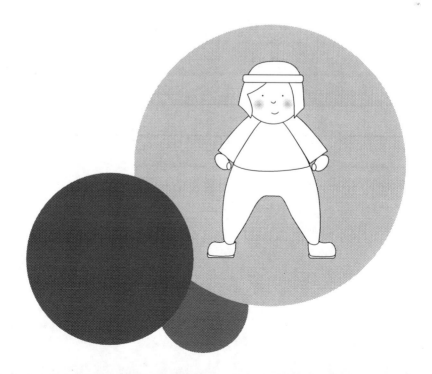

SYNOPSIS

We are all "Fighting Gravity" everyday of our lives. As we move through time and become seasoned individuals, "Fighting Gravity" becomes a difficult challenge. Standing up straight, not gaining extra weight, exercising three days a week minimum and keeping your sense of humor makes aging not for sissies.
We don't need another fitness book trying to make us into 30 year old, body beautiful, human specimens. What we do need is a humorous, self help, fitness book for the 65% of people who don't exercise. We do need a logical, easy, equipment free, positive approach to "move it or lose it." How do we begin a fitness program that is safe, relatively pain free and still have a good time? The motto here is "Just Suit Up and Show Up." Draft your friends who will stick by you during this glorious but sometimes trying experience. Learn to exercise at work, in your car or truck, while on vacation or on your bed. Use objects around the house like stairs, front door or water bottles to promote fitness. Collect points and a "Yea for You" each time you do something positive. The end result will be a new you, feeling and looking better, taller, improved breathing and stronger muscles. You will earn an "Extended Warranty" on your body parts. "Fighting Gravity" is the book you will want to give to your friends, family members and other loved ones to motivate them to fight gravity with you.

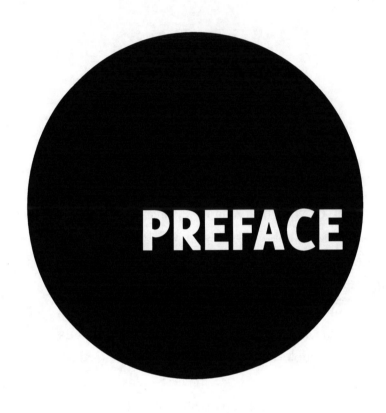

PREFACE

In the 1980's and '90's older people were sometimes called the invisible generation. I'm not talking about "old" old. Not "Mamie Eisenhower, boy she was a hot tamayta" old. I'm talking about people in their 50's and 60's. Pups still, for those of us who are at that age now. But back then many powerful aspects of society (read: advertising and Hollywood) dictated "things are only good as long as you are young" mentality.

The legendary rock group, The Who, declared in their rebellious song, *My Generation*: "Hope I die before I get old" (which I find amusing now that they're in their 60's and still performing that song on tour – but I digress).

That was the kind of attitude the country embraced at the time. In many of the commercials and movies I watched, once you were past 40 things slid down hill. Once you were 50 you were decrepit. And once you got past 60, you became nonexistent. We were a world sold on youth, and as we aged we became aesthetically challenged.

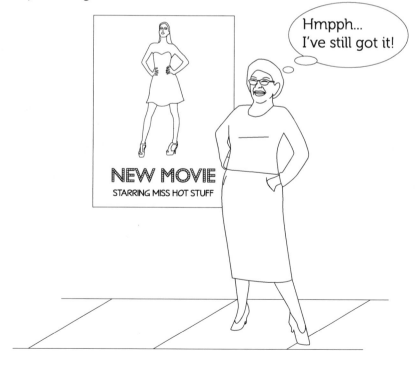

What is "old" anyway? When you really think about it, it is all just an attitude, right? Teenagers look at their parents and think: "Man, 40 is old," while those of us who are at or above that age all know better. I am 64 years old and am more active today than any of my much younger friends. I'm an avid marathon runner, triathlete, and tournament tennis player. In fact I'm one of just a handful of people who have run a marathon on every continent. So I know what I'm talking about. I've never felt better and I still have a lot more energy, strength and enthusiasm left in me.

Fortunately, during the last decade the "getting old stinks" attitude faded away. You can thank one particular phenomenon for that – we baby boomers began to hit our golden years. For all of us born between the years of 1946 and 1964, our fifth and sixth decades are nigh. In fact recent data indicate that 10,000 baby boomers turn 50 every single day. Other reports put it in even more mind-boggling terms:

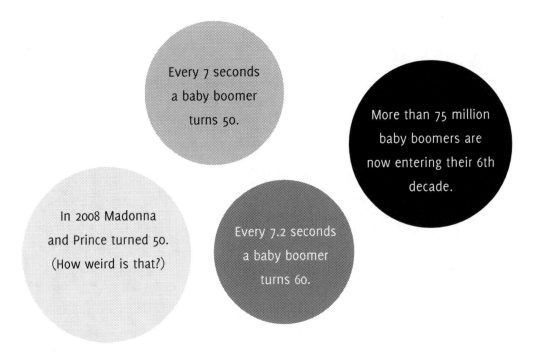

Every 7 seconds a baby boomer turns 50.

More than 75 million baby boomers are now entering their 6th decade.

In 2008 Madonna and Prince turned 50. (How weird is that?)

Every 7.2 seconds a baby boomer turns 60.

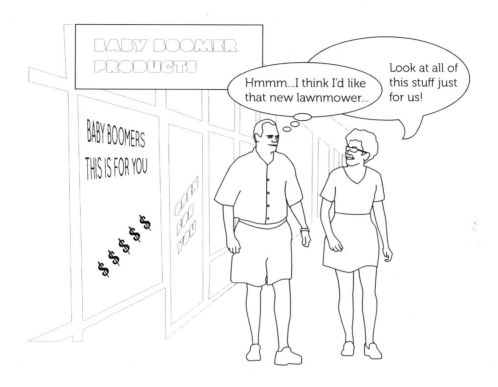

Oh yeah, there's also this interesting little factoid about the boomer generation: We are the single greatest economic force in the country with a combined spending power of $2 trillion.

Money means power and certain aspects of today's society (read: advertising and Hollywood) know when to milk a cash cow when they see it. Now "growing old" is chic and there are marketing campaigns galore aimed at us for products that we'd never had marketed to us before (at least not on the grand scale that they are now): cosmetics, high-tech, and sex (thank you Vitamin V), just to name a few.

We're also changing the face of exercise.

We were the people who were there when the fitness craze started in the 1970's. Remember Jane Fonda? She is making a comeback with exercise videos that are

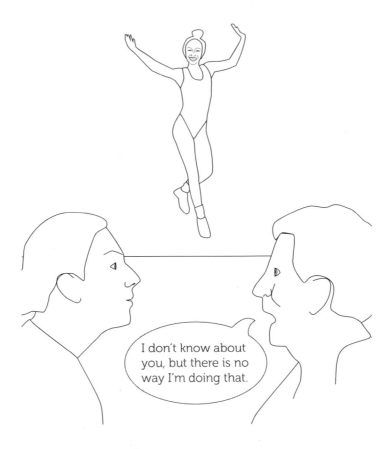

senior friendly. Remember jazzercise? We were an active generation then (grief, we were an activist generation then) and there is no reason to stop. Many health and fitness clubs have already realized the growth of the 55 and over population and are creating special programming for active adults.

However, as we age there may be some adaptations we need to make to ensure that we can stay healthy and avoid injury. Many of us can't take the high-impact pounding of some weight-bearing or cardio exercises that we used to do when we were younger. We need to modify a bit. These modifications affect the way we move and require a little bit of re-education on our body and how we use it. But I guarantee that if you make these changes you will feel more vibrant, more alive and healthier than you have in a long, long time.

I want to motivate **EVERYONE** to be the healthiest and the best they can be by renovating their structure and retrofitting it through proper balance, core strength, alignment of joints, good breathing techniques and simple exercises you can do at home, at work, on a plane – even in your car.

I wrote this book because I have the recipe for extending "the warranty" on your body and I want to share it.

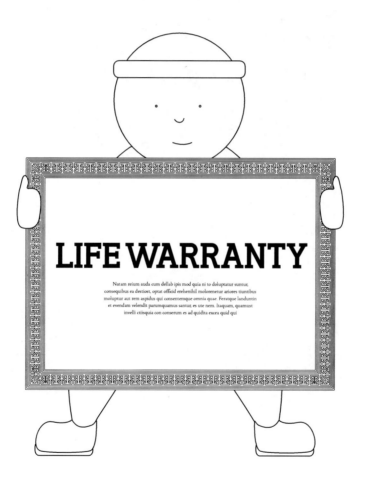

LIFE WARRANTY

Natam reium auda cum dellab ipis mod quia ni to doluptatur suntur, consequibus ea destiost, optat officid erehenihil molorenetur ariores tiuntibus moluptur aut rem aspidus qui consentemque omnia quae. Feratque landuntin et evendam velendit parumquamus santur, es ute nem. Itaquam, quamust invelli ctiisquia con conserum es ad quidita excea quid qui

CHAPTER 1

TERMS AND (DE)CONDITIONS

"OLD HABITS CANNOT BE THROWN OUT THE UPSTAIRS WINDOW. THEY MUST BE COAXED DOWN THE STAIRS ONE STEP AT A TIME."

– MARK TWAIN

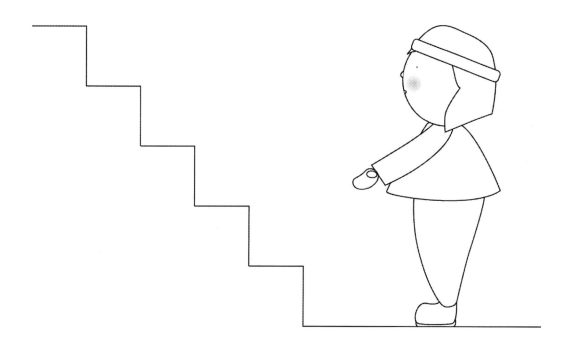

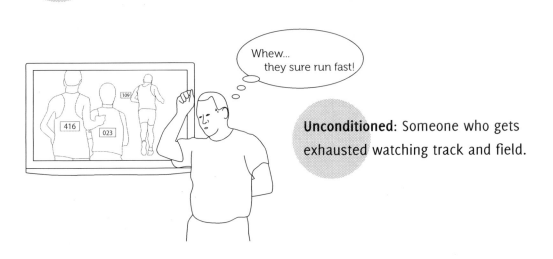

Unconditioned: Someone who gets exhausted watching track and field.

Couch Tomato (female): A professional spectator of TV talk shows.

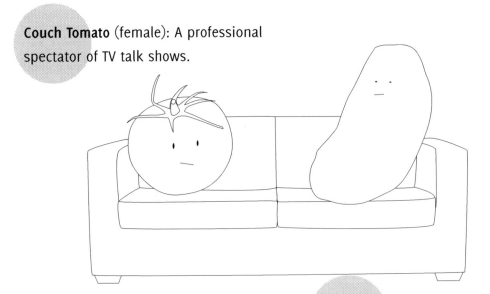

Couch Potato (male): Someone who is gravitationally challenged.

Fit and trim: How all males over 50 see themselves, no matter what. (Especially those you see running or doing yard work without a shirt. Why? Why do they do that?)

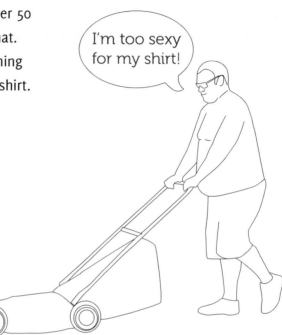

10 lbs overweight: How all women over 50 see themselves, no matter what.

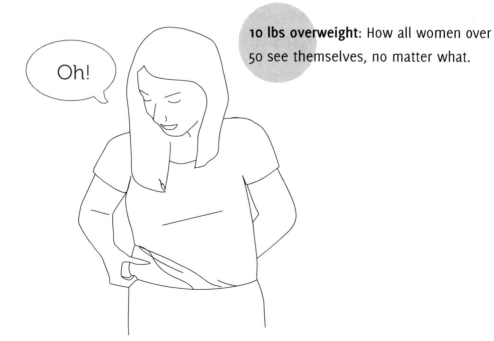

Keesterholic: Someone who's butt has become addicted to vinyl, leather, suede or other forms of chair coverings.

I'm John and my butt is a keesterholic.

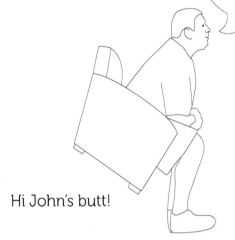

Hi John's butt!

Exercise: Anything other than not moving.

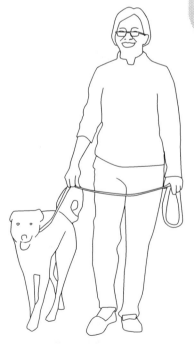

Diet: Chocolate cake, French fries and a Diet Coke.

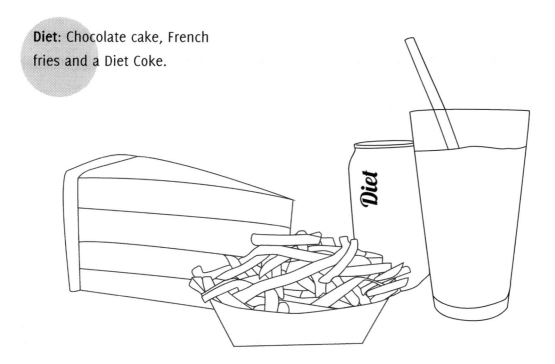

As I mentioned earlier we used to be part of one of the most active demographics in history – the Boomers. When we started the advent of the fitness craze in the 1970's, our credo was "feel the burn". But for many of us that credo has become "hand me the remote." For such an active generation it is a shame that so many of us have stopped enjoying athletic endeavors of any kind.

You know something? Everybody's parts have a shelf life. We don't know exactly what that shelf life is, but I can tell you that one way to prolong the life of your parts is by exercise. And one of the quickest ways to spoil it is simply sitting still.

Why is it that so many of us just stopped exercising? I often ask that question. Sometimes I'll even ask other people. And you know what I hear when I do that? Predominantly these two excuses:

I'm a Sedentary Person and I LIKE It! (a.k.a. I'm OK With My Big Fat Self)

No you aren't, you're just used to it. Not exercising has become a habit. And like any bad habit the longer you keep it up the harder it is to break and the worse the repercussions are. Just like overeating, watching too much TV or belching in public.

A sedentary lifestyle will bring us nothing but harm and the older we get the more dangerous it becomes.

It really comes down to the question of how difficult is it for us to change our habits. For years we have heard the terminology "move it or lose it". That's such an apropos term for all of us, because suddenly we are finding out that the parts we haven't used in 15 years don't work as well. We're not moving them, so now we are losing them.

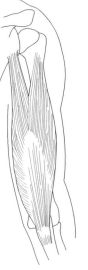 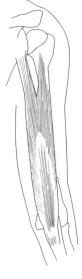

Regular
muscle

Atrophied
muscle

Do you realize that while you're sitting on your sofa or at your desk thinking "boy why does everything hurt?" your muscles are constantly shrinking or atrophying. When your muscles atrophy things start to hurt because your muscles weaken and cannot hold up your bones. What you don't move – you will LOSE. You need to wiggle those parts. Kind of like when your dentist tells you to only floss the teeth you want to keep.

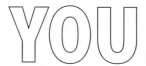

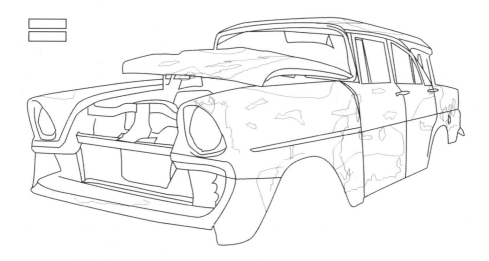

Want another analogy? No? I don't care - this is my book. If you haven't exercised in 13 years your parts are going to be rusty. It is the same if you had a car in the garage for 13 years and then tried to use it. How would it perform? I'm going to go out on a limb and say not well. The battery is dead, the upholstery is torn, tires are flat, and belts are corroded. This is exactly like your body. It, like your car, needs servicing. It needs to be used and maintained in order to keep running.

I know what some of you are saying. Oh, come on, we're not that bad. Not all of us are sedentary or overweight. Maybe not – but it's pretty darn close. Take a look at these little pearls from the official web site of the Surgeon General[1]:

Women gaining more than 20 pounds from age 18 to midlife double their risk of postmenopausal breast cancer, compared to women whose weight remains stable.

Many people live sedentary lives; in fact, 40% of adults in the United States do not participate in any leisure time physical activity.

An estimated 300,000 deaths per year may be attributable to obesity.

Overweight and obesity are associated with an increased risk for some types of cancer including endometrial (cancer of the lining of the uterus), colon, gall bladder, prostate, kidney, and postmenopausal breast cancer.

For every 2-pound increase in weight, the risk of developing arthritis is increased by 9 to 13%.

A weight gain of 11 to 18 pounds increases a person's risk of developing type 2 diabetes to twice that of individuals who have not gained weight.

Over 80% of people with diabetes are overweight or obese.

[1] www.surgeongeneral.gov/library/index.html

The incidence of heart disease (heart attack, congestive heart failure, sudden cardiac death, angina or chest pain, and abnormal heart rhythm) is increased in persons who are overweight or obese.

Less than 1/3 of adults engage in the recommended amounts of physical activity.

Even moderate weight excess (10 to 20 pounds for a person of average height) increases the risk of death, particularly among adults aged 30 to 64 years.

61% of all American adults were overweight or obese in 1999.

Not a pretty picture, huh? It is recommended that Americans accumulate at least 30 minutes of moderate physical activity most days of the week. More may be needed to prevent weight gain, to lose weight, or to maintain weight loss. And according to the figures you just read 40 percent of us are doing nothing at all. Nothing!

To prolong your shelf life you need to stay involved, have interests. At the most rudimentary it's getting out of bed in the morning (which for some is a difficult thing to do), getting dressed and getting out of the house. They may seem like baby steps but they are all part of keeping ourselves going.

So, as NIKE says "Just do it". It doesn't really matter what type of exercise. And you don't need to try to run a marathon right off the bat. Set realistic expectations and build from that. Just a little activity to start the ball rolling and then the sky is the limit. Just 10-15 minutes out of our day can start a whole new lifestyle change. Start doing something. Anything. Set your clock a little early, get

up and walk around the block. One time around the block each day for a week
Then next week walk around the block twice. Get a routine going.

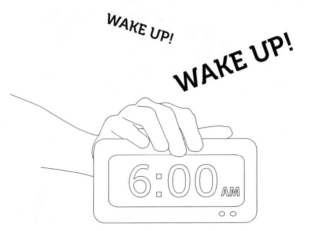

WAKE UP!

WAKE UP!

6:00 AM

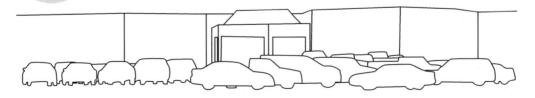

Have a garden? Spend ten
minutes weeding it each day.

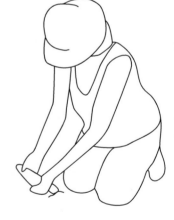

When shopping park your car in the
far corner of the parking lot.

19

Take the stairs instead of the elevator

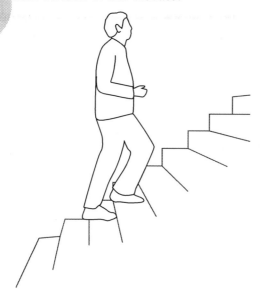

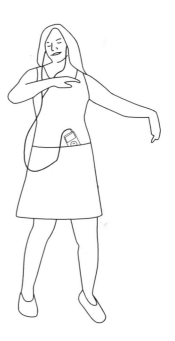

Turn on your radio (or grab your iPod –
sorry, dating myself there) and dance to
a couple of songs in a row.

Just remember – moving is the important thing. Once you get a routine going
you'll be surprised at the results.

Throughout this book I'll be giving you many little informative tidbits on how
you can stay moving it throughout your day – at your desk, driving in a car, even
traveling in a plane. But, first, we have some other things to cover.

I'll Just get Hurt

Back in the late 70's and 80's when we were in our 20 and 30's "Go for the burn" was the physical fitness mantra.

"Let's get physical" sang Olivia Newton John.

John Mellencamp rasped "Hurts so good".

When we were younger that's how we approached physical fitness – and life – for that matter. Pain, shmain – bring it on.

But today we have fears. Maybe it was something along life's path that caused us to rethink not only how we exercise but how we live our lives. Past injuries, failures, emotional turmoil – it could be anything. For crying out loud, just turn on the news any day of the week. If that doesn't turn you gray, I don't know what will. "Life things" have a way to instill fears in many of us.

For many of us it has spread to physical activities. What if it gives me back pain? What if it tears my rotator cuff? What if I get hurt? What if, what if, what if.

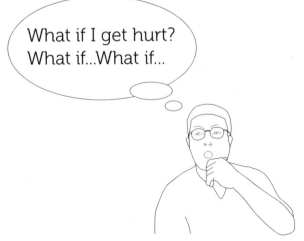

Did you know your chances of getting hurt when you are not exercising can be as great as when you are working out. For example, our hip aches because your butt muscles are weak – it is underuse not overuse.

First and foremost seek advice from your medical doctor before you proceed into a new exercise program. Make sure they know you are going to do something new that has been modified for your needs.

Second, have someone who is knowledgeable in this exercise program tell you BEFORE you begin what you are going to feel like after you start. New sensations can be frightening as we age. You need to have an understanding of what you will be feeling – different muscle sensations, more fatigue etc.

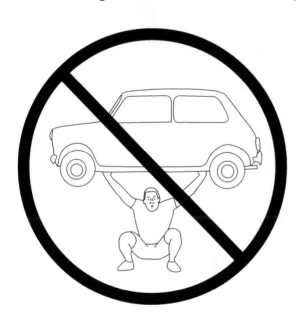

You shouldn't get hurt if your pre-exercise (stretching) program is thorough and your expectations are realistic. Start small, go with a low impact exercise with a small range of motion. As I mentioned earlier don't try running a marathon or lifting a small car. Sounds like common sense. But you'd be surprised how many times I see a de-conditioned person go waaaay too far. My neighbor embarked on a running program after a long lay off. She bought her new shoes and clothes, picked the day to start and out the door she went. Not knowing her endurance level but remembering what it used to be, she just continued to run. When she turned around to run back home, she was so pooped and so far out she had to call me to come get her.

CHAPTER 2

THE "CORE" OF THE MATTER

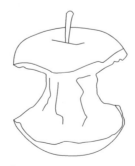

"Snap!

Crackle!

Pop!"

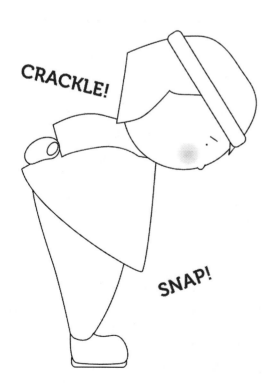

CRACKLE!

SNAP!

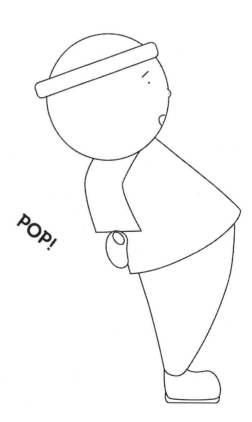

POP!

As I watch people groan as they bend over to pick something up or grimace with each stiff step they take, I can't help but think of a bowl of Rice Crispies, Snap! Crackle! Pop!

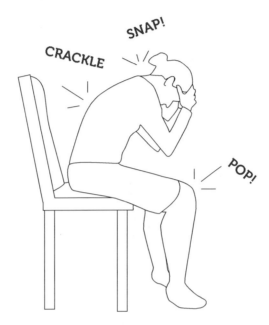

All of the physical pain and suffering that we as human beings endure each day, particularly as we get older, can seem overwhelming at times. Joints are out-of-control painful, muscles cramp more often, and things obviously don't work as well as they did when we were twenty years – or even ten years younger.

It's enough for a person to yell out "Is this it? Is that the best it gets? Am I going to feel this way from now on?!?!"

The answer is a resounding NO.

Good news? But before we get to how we can feel better we need to understand how we got into this physiological mess in the first place.

Most definitely old Father Time has a hand in the increased frequency of stiffness, soreness, cramps, pulls, tears and other anatomical horrors we experience as we get older, but there's another culprit who's even more responsible for this dire state we find ourselves in – ourselves! Wait – that didn't come out right. But does it make sense?

In any event, it should come as no surprise to us that we are the primary reason our bodies betray us. Especially considering what most of us put in our stomachs on a daily basis (I've heard steak has become a top 5 condiment in many Midwestern states) as well as the predominantly sedentary lifestyle many of us choose to lead. But I'm not talking about gluttony, sloth or any other deadly sin right now.

I'm talking about the way we stand, the way we sit, the way we lie down – the way we move and the way we choose to live in our bodies. These are the main

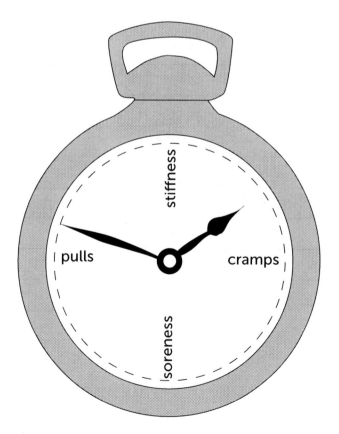

reasons we hurt more than we should as we age. And it's because we learned to move incorrectly as gravity began pulling us toward the pavement.

Huh? you're wondering. I learned to move incorrectly? How can that be? I was born, I started crawling, advanced to the walking stage fairly quickly and have enjoyed the "Golden Age of Mobility" ever since. What's not to like (except my aching back, neck, shoulders, feet, legs, hamstrings, hips and fingers)?

The truth is that we've developed all kinds of bad habits as we've grown that affect the way we move. The most critical one may be the development of our

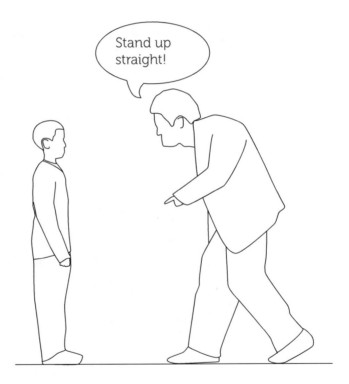

postural alignment. The plain fact is that most of us have bad posture. But it can be corrected – or at least altered for the better – even at this stage of the game.

Now, this is important so listen up. In order to correct bad postural position we need to understand what exactly good posture is. "Stand up straight!" is what our elders were always yelling at us. And, while that may have seemed like solid advice at the time it actually is not the best case scenario for every one.

That's because your spine – the foundation for all things mobile in your body – has four different curves in it – the cervical, the thoracic, the lumbar and sacral. Good posture is making sure that these spinal curves are in alignment with each other when we are walking, running, twisting, turning, etc. When these curves are not in alignment it can put pressure on the spine as well as the front of the

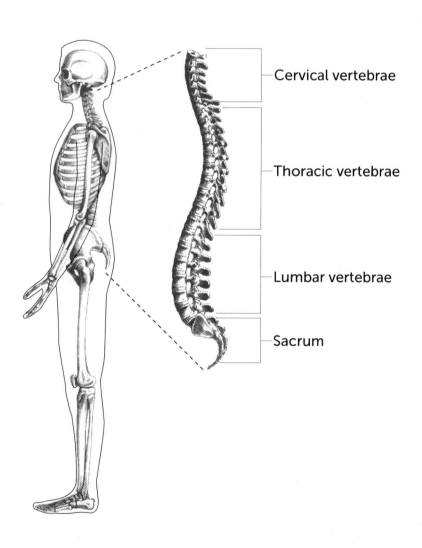

Cervical vertebrae

Thoracic vertebrae

Lumbar vertebrae

Sacrum

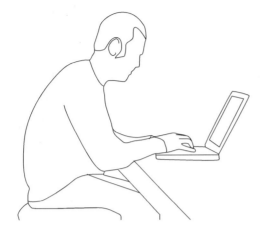

pelvis. Put too much pressure on the muscles and they can become short and tight. Not enough pressure and they can become elongated and weak.

This is what is called a muscular imbalance and it is a leading cause of injury for every type of person in any age group – football players, accountants, dancers, librarians, birthday clowns, whoever. But it is particularly prevalent in the over- 40 crowd. And muscle imbalances aren't limited to the spine, either. They can effect the hamstrings, the shoulders, the neck, the feet – everywhere. It is these imbalances – too much stress on some muscles, not enough on others that can cause tears, pulls, and all sorts of damage.

Now, stay with me here – imbalances in our bodies were caused by the development of poor postural alignment and poor postural alignment is caused by our activities and lifestyle – work activities, leisure activities, social activities. We do many of the same activities each day – strengthening some muscles and under using others.

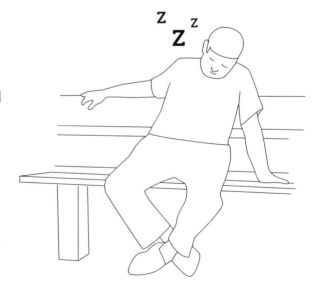

A good example may be how you sit at work. Do you lean forward slightly as you type on your computer? Slump to the same side while you're napping? Lean to the back? All of these positions can contribute to an imbalance as you are straining some parts of your body while ignoring others, causing them to weaken.

So, in many ways how we live dictates our posture. This dictates what kind of muscle imbalances we develop. This dictates the injuries, pain and suffering we find ourselves in.

And now that I've totally bummed you out, it's time for some good news. These muscle imbalances along with the maladies they cause can be eliminated!

That's right! For only $99.99 you too can be cured of all of your bodily ailments with Professor Wintroub's Sweet Elixir of Euphoria... just send a self addressed envelope with a check or money order to...

OK, just kidding there. Yes, I know it may sound like snake oil, but it really isn't.

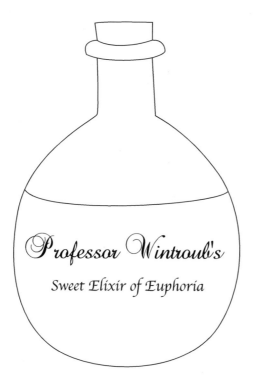

In fact it makes perfect sense. If you learned to move incorrectly, well, you just need to correct your incorrectednes... your incorrectability...your.. uh.. Well, basically you need to learn how to move the right way.

In most of our activities we use our extremities first. Think about how you move. Oops, you just dropped your purse or wallet. What do you do? You lean over at the waist, stretch out your arms and pick it up. Do you know what kind of havoc that wreaks? It puts inordinate pressure on our spine and butt muscles and the muscles and tendons of our arms, neck and legs. That's called moving from the outside (extremities) to the inside (core and abdominal muscles). We need to move from the inside out.

Have you ever caught a guy on the beach sucking in his stomach to impress a pretty girl walking by? You know what? He should be sucking in his stomach. We all should. If your posture is aligned your stomach muscles are working all the time. Good posture actually keeps your core turned on It's part of learning how to use your core to move.

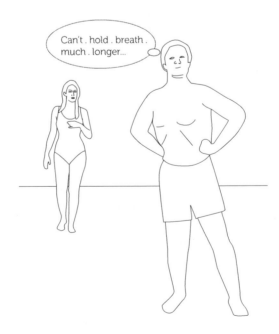

Look what Joseph Pilates – the inventor of the now famous exercise method – had to say on the subject in this excerpt from a 1962 interview in *Sports Illustrated*.[1]

NOTE: Keep in mind that many times Mr. Pilates could be very, um... passionate about his way of thinking. And his opinion toward the American way of life at that time was less than stellar:

"...Americans. They want to go 600 miles an hour and they don't know how to walk! Look at them all in the street. Bent over. Coughing! Young men with gray faces! Why can't they look at the animals? Look at a cat. Look at any animal. The only animal that doesn't hold in its stomach is the pig. Look at them all out on the sidewalk now, like pigs.

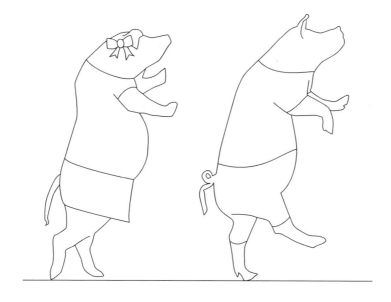

"By exercising your stomach muscles you wring out your body, you don't catch colds, you don't get cancer, you don't get hernias. Do animals get hernias? Do animals go on diets? Eat what you want, drink what you want. I drink a quart of liquor a day plus some beers, and smoke nearly 15 cigars."

Okaaaay, so maybe Joe went a little overboard on all of the benefits of core strength. But keep in mind he did live his life in the way he described.

Here's another analogy of why a strong core is critical that may be simpler for you to understand.

[1] "To Keep in Shape: Act Like an Animal," Sports Illustrated, February 12, 1962.

BODY RETROFITTING

I lived in the Los Angeles area during the 1984 Los Angeles earthquake when so many homes, buildings and other structures collapsed. The damage was enormous. But you know what? People wanted to rebuild. So they did. You can too. You can rebuild the dwelling otherwise known as your body.

Retrofitting your home is the same as retrofitting your body. Once you get the foundation (your core) squared away you can begin to work on the windows and doors and walls. Start with the inside of your body which includes the core abdominal muscles, the diaphragm breathing muscle, the pelvic floor muscles and the small muscles attached to the bones in your back. Then move to the outside large muscles: biceps, triceps, glutes, quads, etc. These muscles when strong work to control your bones and joints.

What would you do first to the house in the picture? Paint? Re-roof? I don't think so.

When your mechanic tells you that you need new tires because the old ones have worn out unevenly and are now dangerous, you immediately get the tires. Would you even consider not balancing the tires before you put them on? No! Why do you take better care of your car than your body?

The point is, a strong core equals a strong body. It will allow you to move the way you are supposed to, exercise the way you are supposed to, live the way you are supposed to. Let's get those body parts aligned, posture improved and frame strengthened.

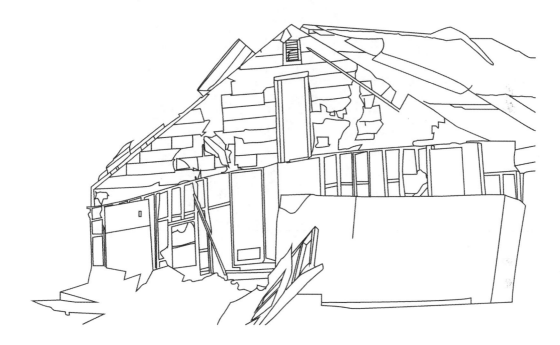

CHAPTER 3

LOOK AT YOURSELF: DO I HAVE TO?
(MIRROR MIRROR ON THE WALL...)

"HAVE YOU LOOKED AT YOURSELF? I MEAN REALLY LOOKED AT YOURSELF?"

– DENISE VENETTI

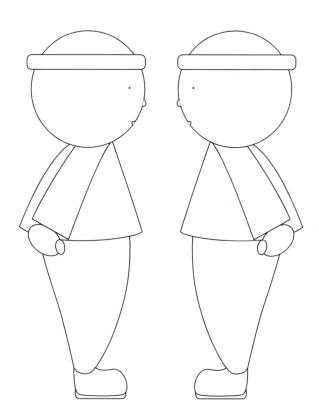

Back in the late '80's on Saturday Night Live comedienne Nora Dunn had a semi-regular character, Denise Venetti, who hosted a psycho-babbling TV self-help show called "Learning to Feel". Guests would come on her show and explain their myriad of problems to Denise who would always be listening intently, hands in a prayer formation resting on her chin, nodding slowly. Her advice to the guests was always the same – she would lean forward and ask earnestly: "Have you looked at yourself? I mean really looked at yourself?"

Every guest would then see the light. "Thank you doctor, I feel so much better!" It didn't matter what the problems were – infidelity, bankruptcy, murder. It was all the same thing. They were all cured by the magic words "Have you looked at yourself?"

Pretty funny stuff.

In the real world looking at yourself can't cure all ills, but an external glance can be a pretty big eye opener with regard to posture and joint placement.

Here's a little exercise you can do when no one is looking that will give you a good idea where you are supposed to be. Be prepared – it can be a little shocking.

THE MIRROR NEVER LIES

First, find a full length mirror to allow viewing your front, back, and sides. Pretend there is a straight line drawn from top to bottom of the mirror, I call the line longitudinal line like on a globe. Now, take off your clothes down to the bare minimum. No really – I said to do this when no one was looking. Once you stop laughing (or gasping, or recoiling) at what you see, let us evaluate the damage life has bestowed upon your poor framework.

37

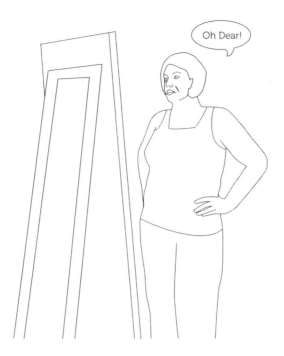

Turn one side toward the mirror and look at the placement of your head, also known as the 8 pound bowling ball at the top of your body. The ball should be sitting directly on top of the cylinder called your neck. Your ear should be above the middle of your shoulder.

So what does all of this mean?

Well, the line on the mirror represents optimal posture, or what your skeleton should look like if your muscles weren't waging a war inside of you. Under your skin, picture several lopsided tugs-of-war happening at the same time. The stronger side keeps pulling on the weaker side like the stronger muscles of your body pull on the bones until they are moved away from the center line on the mirror that you are glaring into. Wild, isn't it?

OK, let's keep looking. Are your shoulders rotating inward? Are they elevated? Are your pinky fingers on the side of your leg or more forward or backward? What do you see?

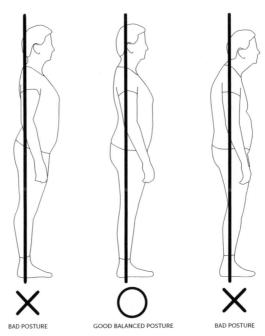

BAD POSTURE   GOOD BALANCED POSTURE   BAD POSTURE

Take a look at your hips. Imagine putting headlights on the front of your hips and taillights on the back. Would the beams point straight ahead? Or would they be askew? Did you know that if your hips are off center this affects your neck and knees? Everything attaches to everything. The thigh bone connected to the hip bone etc.

Play with your hip position a bit by trying to tilt your hips back and forth and see what it does to the rest of your body. If your hips or pelvis point downward try to squeeze your buns together and pull in your navel.

Hard to do, right? When your abdominals and glutes are turned off your body's support system is compromised that means weakness throughout your body. If your car is turned off, it's not going anywhere. If your stove is turned off, it's not cooking anything. If your abdominals and glute muscles are turned off, you look like, Frosty the Snowman. As you can see the alignment of your body parts is a key issue. The goal is to get both sides to match, and then strengthen both sides equally.

39

Don't' be discouraged – identifying the problem is the first step toward fixing it, right?

Next are the ankles. Look for the placement of your ankle bones in alignment with your shoulder. After reviewing the right side do the same with the left. The next part is more difficult. Look at the front view of your framework. Do an evaluation of your body on the line with the mirror. Are your ears even? Is your chin directly above your chest bone (sternum)? Or is your chin pointed right or left? Where are your shoulders?

Try to take an accurate account of your parts without having an emotional involvement (or breakdown). You won't be able to see your backside unless you have a 3-sided mirror and I doubt that you want to invite someone over to assist you with a rear view evaluation. Let's just make the assumption that based on what you have already seen on the first 3 sides that your framework on the back side isn't much better.

I know, this can be somewhat sobering. You are wondering what in the world happened to you while you were busy with life and not paying attention to what was going on under your clothing. John Lennon once said "Life is what happens while you're busy making plans." Sometimes your body has a plan all its own.

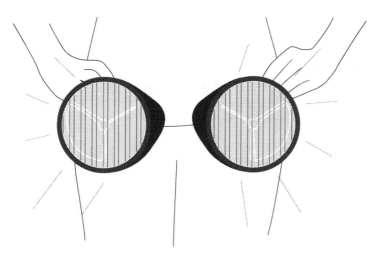

CHAPTER 4

GETTING STARTED
(SUIT UP AND SHOW UP)

"JUST SUIT UP AND SHOW UP"

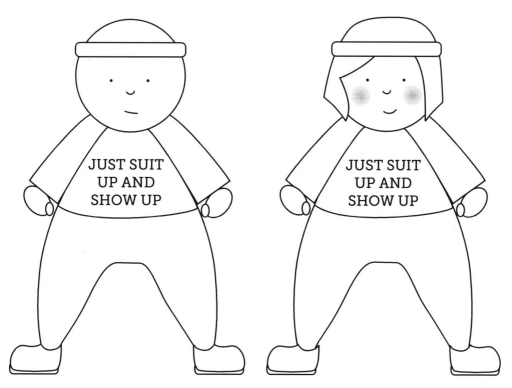

Misery loves company, very negative but true. If you are going to put yourself through this coming out or new you situation I'm sure you would love at least one of your friends to "enjoy" this journey with you. Actually, the more the merrier. Ever see those commercial for osteoporosis medication? There is always four women walking, or doing weights, or some form of exercise in a group. Even the drug companies or is it the advertising agencies believe at least four friends is an appropriate number? Anyway, grab whoever is ready, willing, and able to join you. Since this is going to be a work in progress the journey needs to be fun, enjoyable, and pleasant so don't choose poopy people. When you are too tired to motivate them, they need to motivate you. That is why four is a good number so one is always ready to pull the pack along like in the Tour de France. One rider pulls the pelaton along then one rider replaces him and so on. Try to find a motto, print shirts. Do whatever is necessary to keep the pelaton motivated.

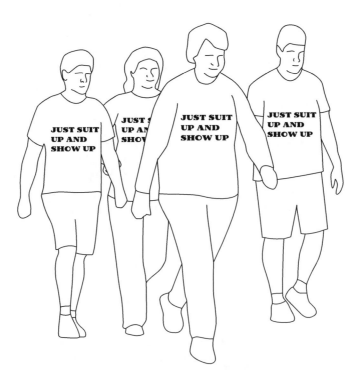

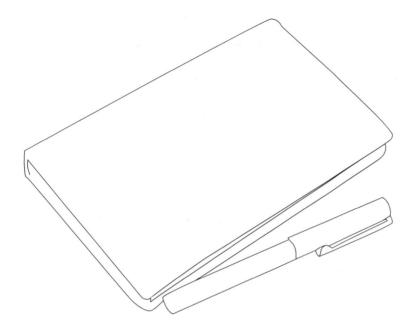

I always liked the motto "Just suit up and show up." I had a friend and buddy athlete who became very ill. But he thought that no matter how badly he felt, if he would "just suit up and show up" he would participate. I have used the term for myself many, many times throughout the years. Choose your own motto or use mine – just get one.

Here are a few suggestions. Each person gets some kind of a diary. It could be just a plain notebook from the drugstore or you could get a Sierra Club calendar notebook from the bookstore. Write in the book everyday even if you don't exercise. Tell the book how you are feeling, what you are eating, how much exercise you are getting. The book is your best friend. It is truly interesting at the end of the year to read through how the past year was for you. You might learn that when you eat a lot of sugary or fatty foods you feel sluggish. Or, after you exercise you feel wonderful for part of the day. Read the book at the end of each week to see what good things happened to you.

As you are exercising see if you and your friends can keep the conversation always positive. Some of my older clients say that getting together with older friends is difficult because the conversation can easily turn to who is sick and who has died. What a fun evening that should be. So they limit the obituary and illness segment to only 5 minutes. That should hold true for you and your exercise buddies. Limit negative thoughts. If you are out for a walk or even mall walking, look for all the exciting things that catch your eye. Find them, they are there.

Just like the song says "lean on me." Everyone needs a helping hand once in a while. Let's say you had a bad case of the flu this year or maybe it just looks miserable outside and you have lost your motivation to move any part of your body. That is when the buddy system really kicks in. your friend or friends need to find the right words or something to coerce you out of the "blue funk" and get you back on track. Sometimes a sweet treat has to be used to get you going again, but you will exercise it off your thighs. No exercise no treat, it worked with Pavlov and his dog, why not you.

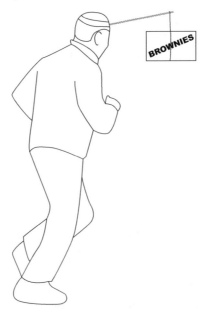

Finally, make a plan and try your hardest to stick to your plan. Here's a plan: exercise every Monday, Wednesday, and Friday at the same time each day. No one is always available all the time, but if everyone knows that "team practice" is 3 days a week at the same time you can schedule your appointments around it.

So let us recap what we have:

- Enlist a friend or friends.

- Find a motto or use "just suit up and show up".

- Make a plan.

- Chart plan in your diary.

- Have a sweet treat ready as a motivational tool.

Okay, now you are ready for take off.

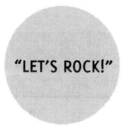

"LET'S ROCK!"

CHAPTER 5

MOVE IT OR LOSE IT EXERCISES
(FIND IT! FEEL IT! USE IT!)

"A BEAR, HOWEVER HARD HE TRIES, GROWS TUBBY WITHOUT EXERCISE."

- A.A. MILNE

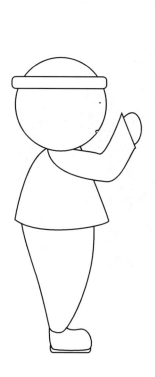

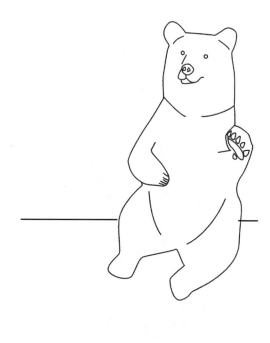

Now that we've talked about why exercising and creating a strong core is so important, here are some simple exercises you can do at home to get those body parts moving and strengthened.

Some of these movements can be done standing, on all fours (quadruped), seated or supine with bent knees (that means on your back). Some are better either standing or seated or supine. I will designate which positions are best. Remember, these movements and exercises are meant to wiggle your parts, oil your joints and make you feel good. You should stop or avoid everything that hurts your back, neck, shoulders or feels as if someone is poking you with a screwdriver.

Do these in sequence when starting. As you get stronger you can mix it up a little bit.

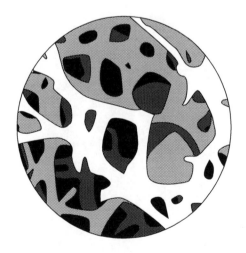

NORMAL BONE DENSITY

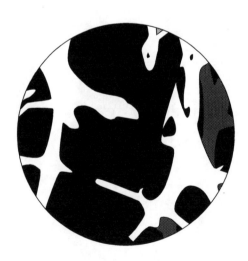

POROUS BONE CAUSED BY OSTEOPOROSIS

BEFORE YOU START – A QUICK NOTE ON OSTEOPOROSIS

Osteoporosis[1], or porous bone, is a disease characterized by low bone mass and structural deterioration of bone tissue, leading to bone fragility and an increased susceptibility to fractures, especially of the hip, spine and wrist, although any bone can be affected.

Osteoporosis is a major public health threat for an estimated 44 million Americans, or 55 percent of the people 50 years of age and older.

In the U.S., 10 million individuals are estimated to already have the disease and almost 34 million more are estimated to have low bone mass, placing them at increased risk for osteoporosis.

Of the 10 million Americans estimated to have osteoporosis, eight million are women and two million are men, showing that 80% of those affected by osteoporosis are women.

If you are over the age of 40 and beginning an exercise program, consult with your physician about osteoporosis. There are several tests available that can let you know if you have it or are a prime candidate to get it. If you do have osteoporosis make sure you talk to your doctor to see what type of exercise movements you should avoid.

OK – let's go.

[1]http://www.nof.org/osteoporosis/diseasefacts.htm

THE HIP DANCE

Position: Standing, Seated, Quadruped, Supine with bent knees

Repetitions: 3-5 times

Remember shimmy fringe on Goldie's outfits on Laugh In, the twist and the hula hoop? Let's see if those aging hips still move to and fro. This movement isolates your pelvis from the rest of your body and it is not easy.

1. Put your hands on your hipbones.

2. Gently rock your hips forward and backward without using your chest, your head or your shoulders.

3. Your beams should be able to point down toward the floor, up toward the ceiling or straight ahead depending upon your hip position.

No matter what position your body is in, your hips and pelvis should be able to move. Do these movements slowly so you can feel how they work and where they come from within your body. Once you can picture the flashlights beams pointing straight ahead you are ready to move on.

Helpful Hint: Imagine say there are flashlights with the beams on and they are tied to the front of your hipbones just like the headlights on a car.

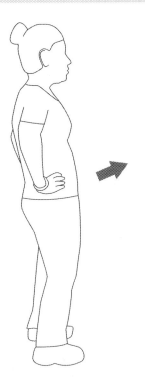 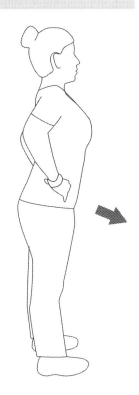

STOMACH SANDWICH

Position: Standing, Seated, Supine with bent knees

Repetitions: 3-5 times

1. Place one hand palm side down on your navel.

2. Place the other hand palm up on the small of your lower back (lumbar spine) – this is what I call a "stomach muscle sandwich."

3. Inhale deeply.

4. As you exhale say "S" to force your diaphragm to help push the air out of your lungs (This flattens your navel, tightens your deep stomach muscles (the transverses abdominis) and secures your deep back muscles (the multifidi)).

5. Tighten or squeeze your pelvic floor called a Kegel. Then imagine you are squeezing a $100 bill between your buns (insert your own joke here). Your pelvic floor is a muscle that acts sort of like a like a trampoline and basically holds your stuff inside of your body.

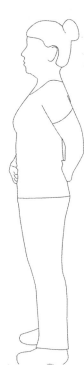

Make sure those beams don't move during the following exercises – just like your car when it turns right or left and the headlights point ahead.

Helpful Hint: it's not necessary to squeeze your pelvic floor tightly when you are doing abdominal exercises, so as you breath out, pull your navel in and tighten your pelvic muscles. Notice that your "headlights" didn't move.

THIGH PRESS

Position: Seated, Supine with bent knees

Repetitions: 3-5 times each leg

1. Place your right hand just above your right knee.
2. Press on the thigh, feeling your deep abdominal muscles tighten.
3. If lying supine do not flatten your lower back to the floor. Remember to use your stomach muscle.
4. Let your navel fall into your spine but don't move your hips.
5. Alternate left hand to left thigh, and right hand to right thigh.

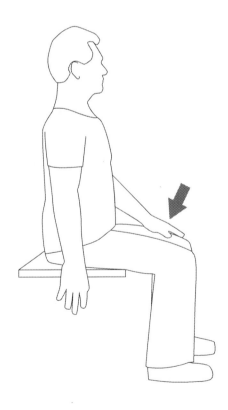

BUN AND CHEST BURNER

Position: Seated, Supine with bent knees

Repetitions: 3-5 times each side

1. Place your right hand on the outside of your right leg.

2. Press your leg against your hand without any movement. See if you can activate your chest muscle and your bun muscle.

3. Alternate from your left side then to your right side.

* For all these exercises on the following pages, inhale to prepare then exhale for a count of five, pulling in on your navel.

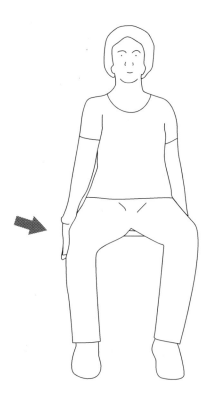

BACK AND SHOULDER BURNER

Position: Seated, Supine with bent knees

Repetitions: 3-5 times each side

1. Place your right fist on the inside of your right knee and press your knee against your fist.
2. Lower your armpit and slide your scapula into your right back pocket.
3. Alternate hands and thighs.

These movements are meant to awaken your parts and prepare you for the following exercises.

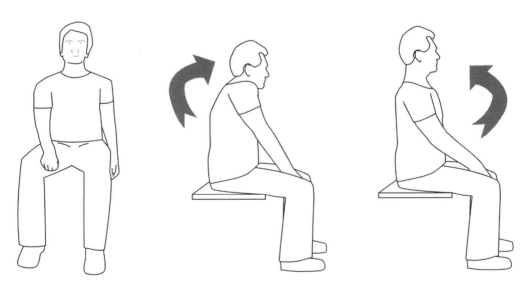

RIB CAGE BREATH

Position: Standing, Seated, or supine with legs bent

Repetitions: 3-5 times

1. Place two fingers from your right hand on your right nostril as you lean to the right.
2. Inhale to feel the rib cage on your left side expand.
3. Take your fingers away from your nose to exhale.
4. Alternate sides to get the feeling of rib cage expansion on the sides and the back of your body. This is called posterior lateral breathing.

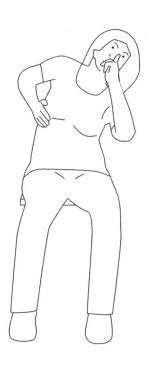 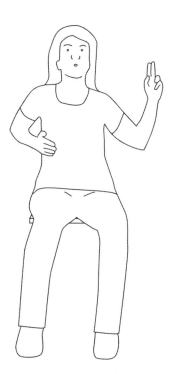

RIBCAGE ARMS (PUPPET ARMS)

Position: Seated, standing or supine with legs bent

Repetitions: 5 times each arm

1. Bring your arms in front you with your fingers pointing forward or toward the ceiling if you are lying down.
2. Start with the right arm and lengthen your right arm making your right arm grow longer than your left arm.
3. Pull your shoulder back where it started without bending the elbow.
4. Alternate arms.

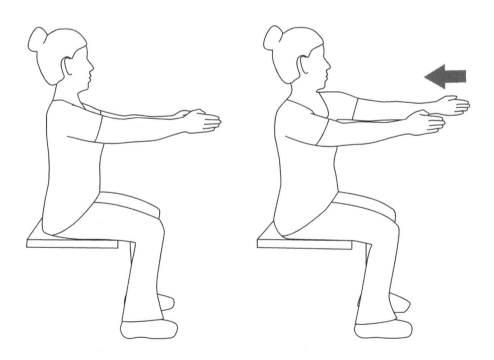

ANGELS IN THE SNOW (OR SAND)

Position: Standing or supine with straight legs

Repetitions: 3-5 times

Did you ever make a snow angel as a kid (or a sand angel if you were from Southern California)?

1. Move your arms slowly upward and downward as if you were making angel wings in the snow.

2. Relax your neck and shoulders, making sure that no other body parts move while your arms are moving.

3. Move your legs open and close (supine position).

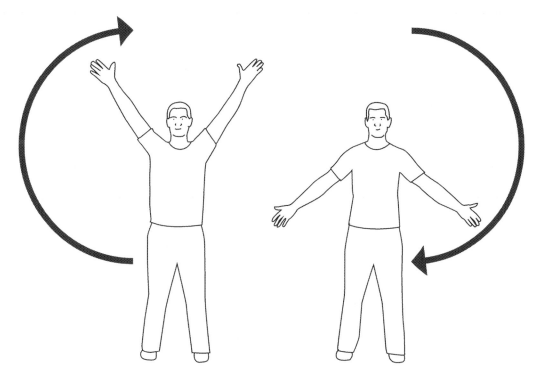

For the next three exercises our motto will be "your back is only as strong as your abdominals."

These movements need to be done using the "stomach muscle sandwich" position and your "headlight beams" pointed toward the ceiling.

LEG FLOATS

Position: Supine

Repetitions: 3-5 times each leg

1. Float your right leg off the floor as if a helium balloon is pulling your leg to a table top position.
2. Slowly return the right foot to the floor.
3. Repeat with the other leg.
4. Do not flatten your back into the floor.
5. Practice these movements until you feel as if your abdominals are controlling your leg movements.

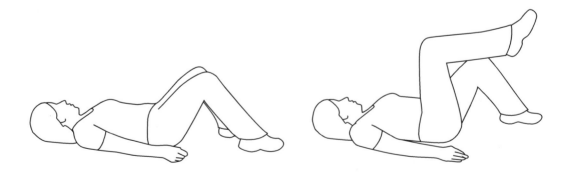

TOE TOUCHES

Position: Supine

Repetitions: 3-5 times each leg

1. Barely lift your right foot off the floor.

2. As you lower your right foot raise the left.

3. Alternate legs.

4. Make sure your stomach muscle sandwich is working, your "beams" are pointed to the ceiling , no stress in your lower back and pain free.

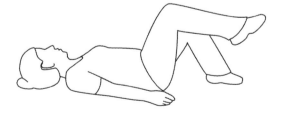 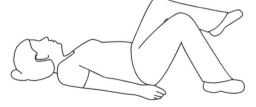

FOOT SLIDES

Position: Supine

Repetitions: 3-5 times each leg

1. Slide one foot out on the floor as far as you can control holding your stomach muscles tight and return the foot before starting the other leg.
2. Gradually extend the leg straight out.
3. Alternate legs.

SAFETY TIP: Remember – these movements are to strengthen your deep abdominals. These exercises can hurt your lower back if you arch your back when you do the movements.

Helpful Hint: Make the range of motion small at first. If you are having trouble sliding your foot out on your own, use a paper plate under your foot to help it slide.

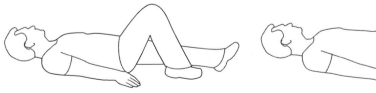

THE BUN BRIDGE

Position: Standing, Supine

Repetitions: 3-5 times each leg

NOTE: You can stand on one leg when you are waiting in line anywhere. This weight bearing exercise helps to strengthen the bun muscles.

1. In supine position lift your buns off the floor about five inches.
2. Squeeze the buns as if you were trying not to drop a $100 bill.
3. Place your hands under your buns to hold them up, remove your hands and feel your bun muscles contract or "fire."
4. Remember your hip joints are only as strong as your bun muscles surrounding the joints. When this movement becomes easy, then do your "toe touch movements" while your buns are in the air.

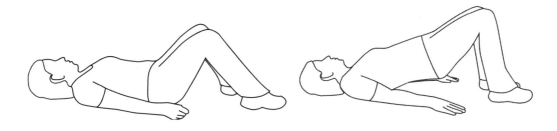

THE BUN SQUEEZE

Position: Seated

Repetitions: 3-5 times

1. Squeeze that imaginary $100 bill while seated, until you poop out the bun muscles.
2. Repeat until you feel a slight burning sensation in the buns.

Helpful Hint: This is a great exercise as it can be done anywhere – while seated in a movie, in an airplane or in front of the TV.

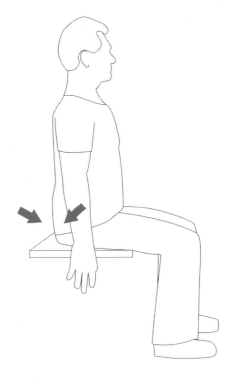

MID-BACK PRESS

Position: Supine with knees bent

Repetitions: 3-5 times each arm

NOTE: You will need a small stack of paper napkins or washcloths for this exercise.

1. Place your arms at your sides palms up, with the stack of napkins or cloths under each hand.
2. Gently press down on the napkins or cloths with your right hand. Hopefully you will feel this movement coming from your upper mid back.
3. Alternate hands.
4. You should also feel the back of your upper arms (triceps) tighten.

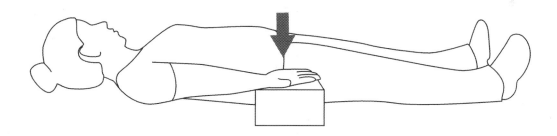

ARM ROTATIONS (CIRCLES)

Position: Standing supine

Repetitions: 3-5 times each arm

1. Turn your palms face up and then face down. See if you can do this movement from your shoulders not your elbows.

2. Make small circles with each arm, palm facing upward as if holding a small candle.

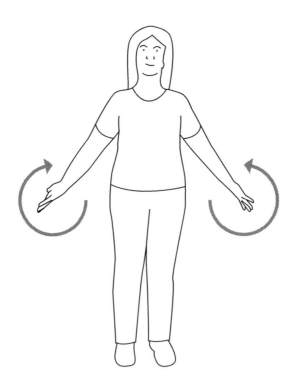

KNEE STIRS

Position: Supine

Repetitions: 3-5 times

The goal here is to warm up the hip glue and move it around in the hip sockets.

1. Bring your right knee into your right hand.
2. Move the knee in little circles as if you were circling the thigh bone (femur) in your hip socket.
3. Circle one direction then reverse.
4. Alternate legs.

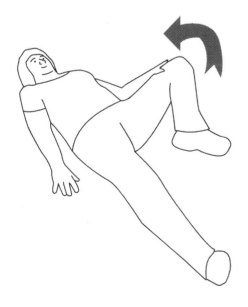 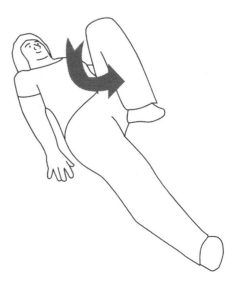

NOSE NOD

Position: Supine with knees bent

Repetitions: 5 times

1. Place your hands behind your head (stop immediately if this causes shoulder pain).
2. Gently elongate the back of your neck using your hands.
3. As you lengthen your neck drop your chin toward your chest and look at your knees.

Helpful Hint: When elongating your neck imagine you are walking with a book balanced on your head. You would lengthen your neck by pushing the book toward the ceiling while not moving your head. That's the feeling you are going for but on the floor in supine with bent knees.

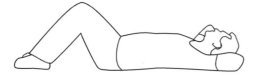
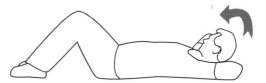

Congratulations on completing all the movements in this chapter.

Continue doing these movements until they become easy – then it's time to move up to the next level.

CHAPTER 6

THE WORKPLACE WORKOUT

PETER: "SO I WAS SITTING IN MY CUBICLE TODAY, AND I REALIZED, EVER SINCE I STARTED WORKING, EVERY SINGLE DAY OF MY LIFE HAS BEEN WORSE THAN THE DAY BEFORE IT. SO THAT MEANS THAT EVERY SINGLE DAY THAT YOU SEE ME, THAT'S ON THE WORST DAY OF MY LIFE."

PSYCHIATRIST: "WHAT ABOUT TODAY?
IS TODAY THE WORST DAY OF YOUR LIFE?"

PETER: "YEAH".

PSYCHIATRIST: "WOW, THAT'S MESSED UP."

- FROM THE 1999 MOVIE, OFFICE SPACE

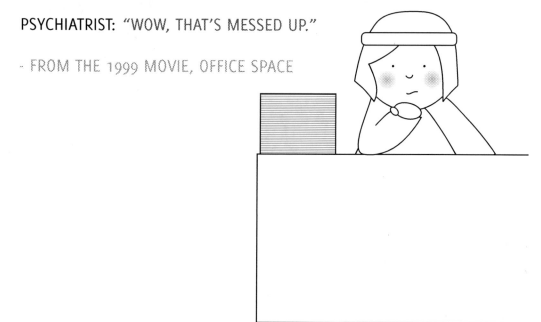

OK, the workplace is not as bad as that. Geez, I certainly hope it isn't. However, it can be a place of pain – physical pain. You wouldn't believe how much damage you can do to your body by sitting at a desk for an extended period of time.

Consider these facts[1]

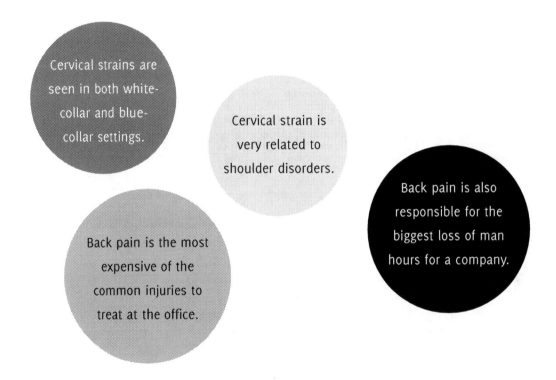

[1]AAHFRP "Ergonomics for the Fitness Professional"

Dynamic muscle energy – the energy you get when you exercise – improves your blood circulation. That's good. Static muscle energy – like when you are sitting at a desk – decreases blood flow, decreases nutrient and waste removal, and requires ten times more energy to recover. That's bad. Basically, sitting at a desk is an absolute killer for the human body.

When sitting at a workstation a good rule of thumb is not too sit for longer than 30 minutes at a time. Even if you have perfect posture sitting for half an hour or more is still going to cause problems. Therefore, you need to be moving every 30 minutes.

Also, if you are staring at a computer screen it is important to look somewhere else other than the screen from time to time to rest your eyes. Staring at a computer screen causes eye-strain that causes issues like blurry vision and headaches.

In addition, your neck, upper back and head can also experience problems due to cumulative trauma or overuse syndrome. At your desk when your head is leaning forward there is pressure on the upper back, the neck and the jaw. It also puts you in a position where there is no support for the weight of the arms. Think about this: each of your arm weighs about 3 pounds and your head is like a 8 pound bowling ball resting on a cylinder called your neck. It creates terrible stress on the body for people who sit at the desk all day.

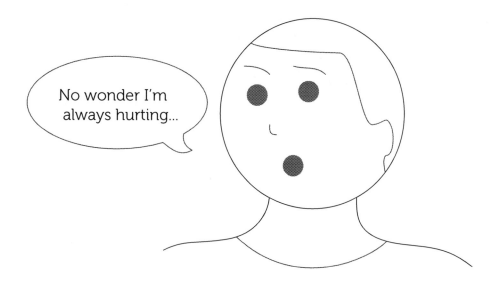

No wonder I'm always hurting...

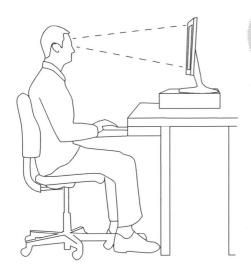

Higher Monitor – Set your computer monitor higher on the desk. You should be able to be in a position where you can sit back on the chair where you can relax your body.

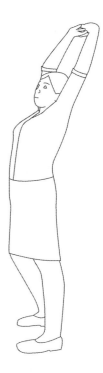

Frequent Stretch Breaks – Get up and stretch every 15 minutes or so. Or lean against the wall and let the wall support your back, head, and arms. Use the wall like a reclining chair.

Put a phonebook under one foot – This will stagger the way your hips are sitting in a chair. Make it so one foot is sitting higher than the other, moving the phonebook to one foot then the other. This helps to unlevel your hips allowing your muscles to lengthen and shorten instead of locking down. Kind of like walking up and down hills instead of walking on a flat surface.

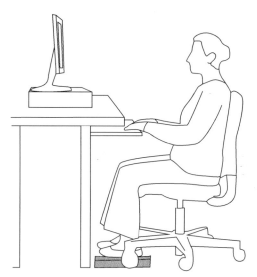

Find an alternative to a chair – There are several inexpensive products now on the market that you can use instead of a standard desk chair. For example:

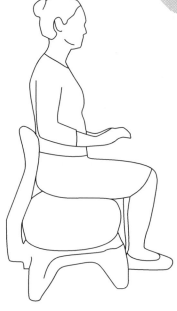

The physioball sits inside of a chair frame making your posture more erect or you can bounce gently on the ball to work your muscles, but it is still important to get up and move around every fifteen to twenty minutes.

Sit/Lean Stool is another comfortable option and it is easy to get in and out of. It's something that you sort of sit and lean against in an almost standing position. This way the weight of the top of your body is not sitting on or compressing the lower part of your body.

Remind yourself to get up and move – One of the things I do in my Pilates studio is give my clients little "happy face" stickers. They put a sticker in their cubicle or office at work – maybe on their desk or computer monitor. The smiley faces are a reminder that they should get up to move around, stand up, walk around their desk – whatever – just keep moving every once in a while.

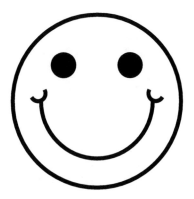

In the 80's corporate fitness was all the rage. This started when many Japanese companies used to line up all their people before they went to work to do a calisthenic program. Then many U.S. companies began to follow suit and offered fitness programs for their employees. Today, with obesity rising as well as the cost of corporate healthcare, many companies are pulling back on fitness programs – it just costs too much for them to keep it going. Now it is up to you.

Here are some simple "desk exercises" you can do to keep the circulation flowing and releave some of that muscular and joint stress while at work.

DESK PRESS

Position: Seated

Repetitions: 3-5 times

Benefit: Strengthens triceps, lats, abs, posture, mid back.

1. Put your arms out in front of you and just press on the desk (are you sitting? standing?). This is works for stomach muscles, triceps, shoulder and other body parts.

2. Cross your right arm to the left side and press down on the desk.

3. Alternate crossing them the other way and repeat the exercise. This works your oblique muscles.

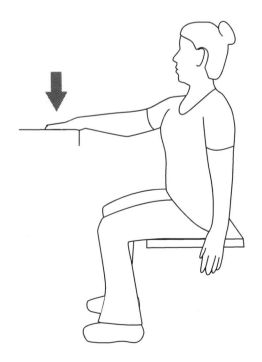
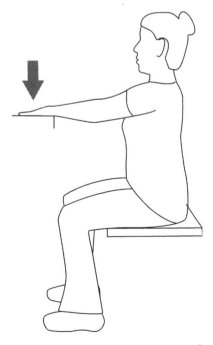

BICEP CURLS

Position: Seated

Repetitions: 3-5 times

Benefit: Strengthens Biceps, Abs and posture muscles.

1. Put your hand under your desk and press like you're trying to lift the desk (you're not actually trying to lift it, Hercules, you're just pressing hard). This is what is known as an isometric bicep curl. Isometric exercises like these are valuable because they really work a specific spot and are "bone-loading", which means the exercises can create more bone density strength than other exercises.

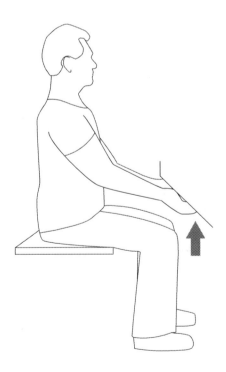

SIT TO STAND

Position: Sitting to Standing

Repetitions: 10 times

Benefit: Buns, quads, abs.

1. Get up from your chair and sit back down.

2. Repeat in sets of 10 throughout the day.

Just by standing up from the chair in neutral pelvic zone you're doing glute and quad work You're also creating strength in your lower body which is good because the longer you sit the weaker your glutes become. They become spongy because they aren't working to hold you up, they are turned off.

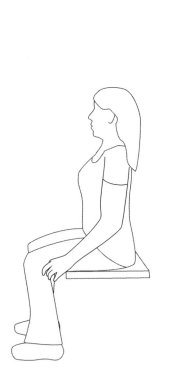
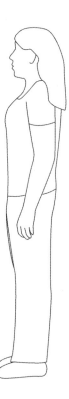

LEG LIFTS

Position: Seated or Standing

Repetitions: 3-5 times

Benefit: hip flexors, posture, balance.

1. While sitting at your desk try to bend your knee up to your nose. Make sure you are not rolling backwards as you are lifting the knee

2. An alternative to this exercise is to stand and march in place as this gets the blood flowing.

By using your legs you are warming up major muscle groups within your body and getting rid of the waste and toxins that accumulate when you are sitting still.

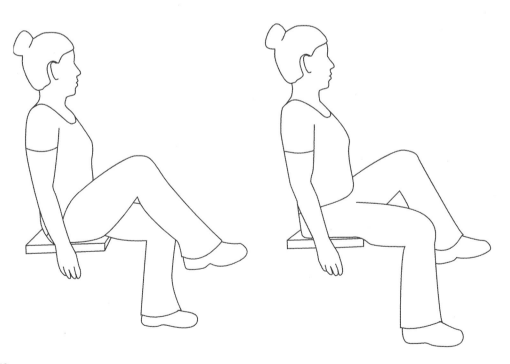

POINT & FLEX

Position: Seated, Standing

Repetitions: 5-10 times

Benefit: Strengthens and stretches lower leg muscles, help posture, balance and ankle flexibility.

1. Go up on your tiptoes and rock back on your heels.
2. This gently stretches your hamstrings and builds up the calf muscles. This is important because as we age we lose the ability to point and flex our feet at the ankles (plantar and dorsiflex) necessary to walk without limping

The ability to do these two moves allow us to keep walking normally. If you lose the ability to point and flex your feet you lose the ability to swing your leg underneath your hip – you have to swing it to the outside, which throws out your back and hips.

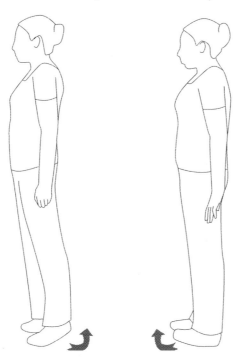

ABDUCTION PRESS

Position: Seated

Repetitions: 3-5 times each leg

Benefit: Strengthens hip joint and bun muscles.

1. Move your chair to one side of the desk, take the outside of one leg and press it against the desk then release the pressure. Hold this isometric exercise for a count of 10 while breathing out and pulling in the navel.

2. Repeat the movement on the other leg.

What this is doing is abduction, or working the muscles on the outside of your leg and more glute work, as wells as rotators for the lower body.

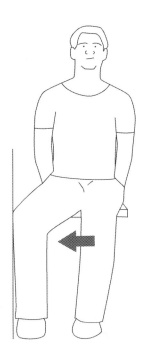

MID BACK & SHOULDER ISOMETRIC PRESS

Position: Seated

Repetitions: 3-5 times each arm, isometric contraction counting to 10 while breathing out and pulling the navel in.

Benefit: Strengthen deltoids and mid back.

1. Make a fist with your hand while you are sitting with your knees bent under your desk.

2. Take your fist and push it against the underside of the desk, and push out and back.

You are working your deltoids and the posterior deltoids. The stronger your back muscles are the more you will be able to hold your head up without eventually straining your neck muscles. That's key. You will be able to lift your arms and hold your head upright by working the mid-back and the deltoid muscles instead of always straining your neck by using neck muscles to lift your arms.,

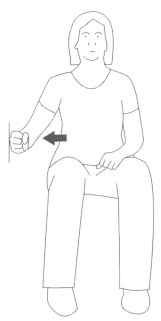

ISOMETRIC PUSH UP

Position: Standing

Repetitions: 3-5 times counting to 10, breathing out while pulling in your naval.

Benefit: Strengthen back and arms.

1. Place your hands on the edge of the desk and pretend you are trying to push your self away from the desk without moving your body.

This works your deep abs and stabilizes your mid-back as your deep abdominals are working to hold you in an upright position. This is a great exercise to strengthen your mid-back since it is always a weak area – particularly for women, who lose upper body strength as well as men who do too many pectoral exercises. This exercise also increases bone density for both the back and the wrists. This becomes crucial as we age because those are the two areas that are affected by osteoporosis.

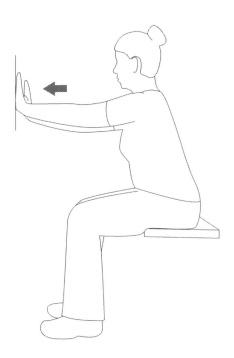

BACK EXTENSION

Position: Standing

Repetitions: 3-5 times

Benefit: Posture, back strengthening, stretching front muscles.

1. Stand behind your chair.
2. Stand on your left leg and point the toe of the right leg behind while you try to lift your chest up to the ceiling (basically, you're trying to slightly bend backward from the tip of your toe to the top of your head to form a crescent moon).

This is what is known as a back extension exercise. It also stretches out the stomach muscles which become "short and tight" because gravity is pulling you toward the floor when you are just sitting at a desk. So a nice stretch through out the day of the front of your body is important because you are getting shorter through the center.

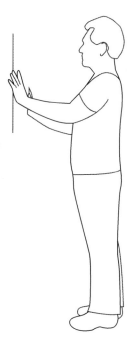 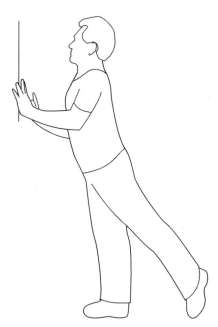

Position: Stand behind your chair

Repetitions: 3 – 5 times

Benefit: Balance and back strengthening.

1. Lift one arm over head extend opposite leg behind you, hold the position for 3 seconds, then switch. Repeat 5 times.

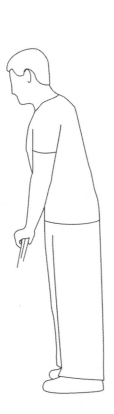
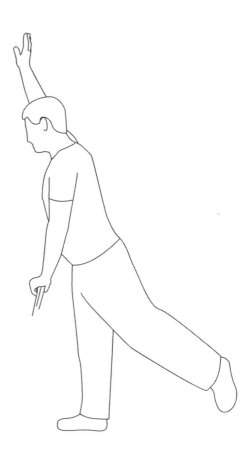

CAN- CAN

Positions: Seated towards front of the chair and sitting up tall.

Repetitions: 3- 5 times

1. Put your toes and knees together and rotate your legs to the left and then back to the right and then left.

2. Extend right leg straight, kicking as you were a can-can dancer and start to the right side and back to the left and right. Extend left leg straight and kick.

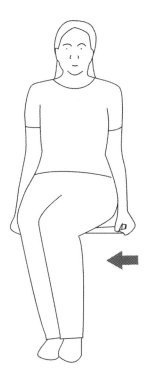
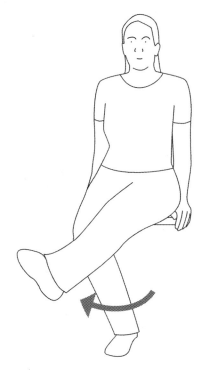

CHAPTER 7

STAYING FIT IN YOUR CAR OR TRUCK

"IT IS THE SPIRIT THAT BUILDS THE BODY."

- FREDRICH SCHILLER.

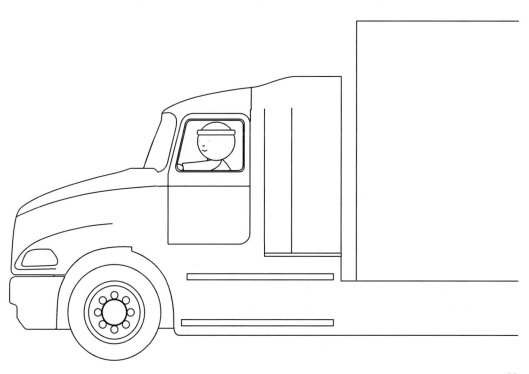

So you have been sitting down at a desk all day; stagnant. You're metabolism is slowing down, you're tired after you eat lunch, and it's a struggle to stay productive. Suddenly it is time for your evening commute. YESSSSS! Could the day get any better? And of course, on the drive home you are stuck in a massive traffic jam. And you find your self in the same position you've been in all day. And you're body begins to ache and cramp just like it did when you were behind a desk.

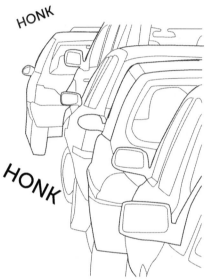

But do not fear - you actually can exercise in the car – even in stop and go traffic – safely. The first thing you can do are breathing exercises. Breathing can relax the weary mind. Keep breathing as in the Pilates 100 exercise moves blood to the organs and brain which can make you more alert.

In your car on your drive home, take a nice big inhale through the nose and exhale through the mouth, making an "S" or hiss sound. After you've done 5 "S" breaths, inhale and open the back of throat and on the exhale say "aaaaaah". Sounds silly, yes, But it is effective. The S-hissing breath helps push the air out of the lungs – when the lungs are empty they fill up deeply when you inhale. Like swimming push all the air out then inhale deeply to fill them up again.

Now you can use your steering wheel for exercises. No, seriously – I wouldn't lie to you. When you come to a stop light, there are many push-pull excercises using your steering wheel that are similar to the desk press in the previous chapter with the steering wheel taking the place of the desk.

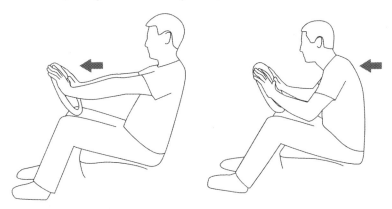

So you are doing upper body exercises. You can rock your pelvis while you are in the car, you can do glute squeezes in the car. Even taking one hand off the steering wheel and pressing on the ceiling as if you are trying to push the roof off (make sure you are at a stop of course) helps keep your scapula depressed (shoulders down, relaxes your neck muscles, armpits lower, gets your neck away from your ears which can relieve neck muscle tension). Put your head against the head rest of your car and do deep breathing. All of these are making you proactive and more alert.

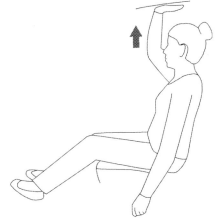

Nope, I haven't forgotten about you truckers out on the road. Here's ten strength training exercises you can do behind the steering wheel of your 18 wheeler – at a rest stop, not while driving. (OK you can actually do these in your car. They just work really well in a truck!)

TIP: Sit up tall when doing each exercise.

Hold the seat with your Right hand, lean forward, pulling your right shoulder backwards. Switch hands and repeat exercise. Use both hands to hold the seat, pinch shoulders back and together. Repeat 3 times.

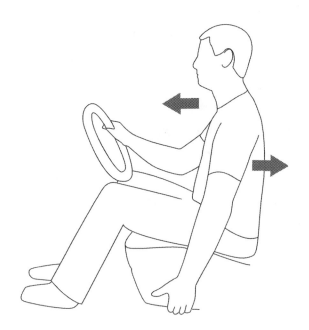

Place both hands on the ceiling of the truck and push against the ceiling while allowing your shoulders to slide downward. Repeat 3 times.

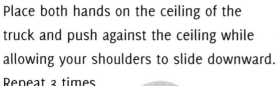

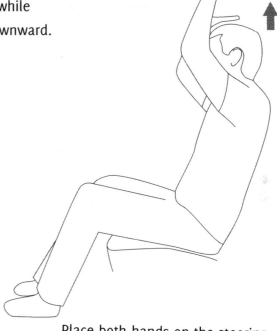

Place both hands on the steering wheel at 3 and 9 o'clock. Pull the steering wheel apart for a count of 10 while exhaling. Repeat 3 times.

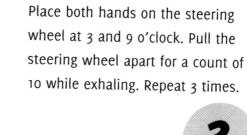

Place both hands on the steering wheel at 3 and 9 O'clock. Squeeze the steering wheel for a count of 10 while exhaling. Repeat 3 times.

4

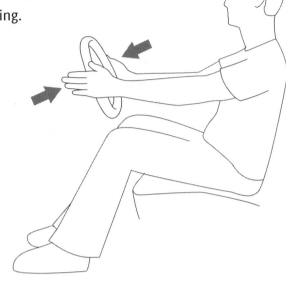

Place both hands on the steering wheel at 3 and 9 O'clock. Push on the wheel as if you were pushing the wheel into the engine for a count of 10 while exhaling. Repeat 3 times.

5

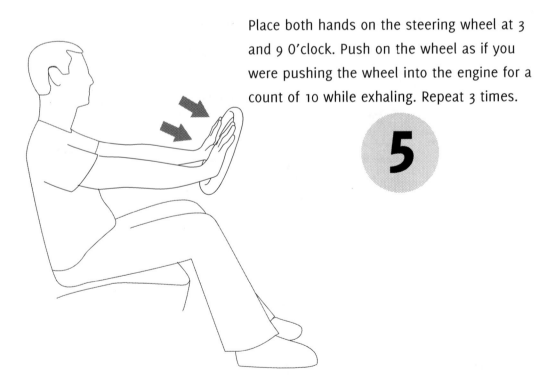

Place hands palms up underneath the steering wheel. Do a bicep curl by trying to pull the steering wheel towards you. Hold for a count of 10 while exhaling. Repeat 3 times.

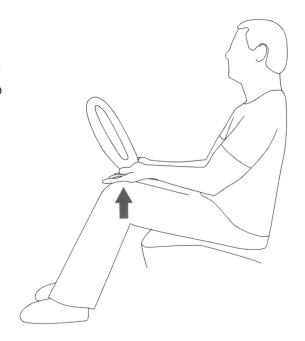

Push your right foot into the floor of the truck while tightening the top of your leg (quadriceps). Hold for a count of 10 while exhaling. Switch legs. Repeat 3 times for each leg.

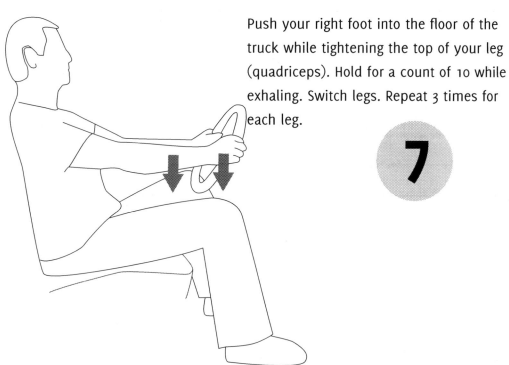

Push your right heel into the floor of the truck. Try to pull the floor towards the seat tightening the back of your leg (hamstrings). Hold for a count of 10 while exhaling. Switch legs. Repeat 3 times for each leg.

8

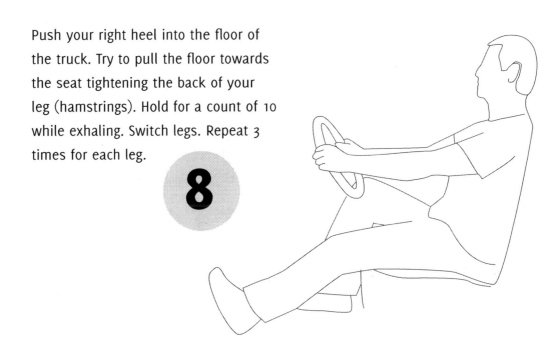

Squeeze your butt muscles together as if holding a 100 dollar bill. Hold for a count of 10 while exhaling. Repeat 10 times.

9

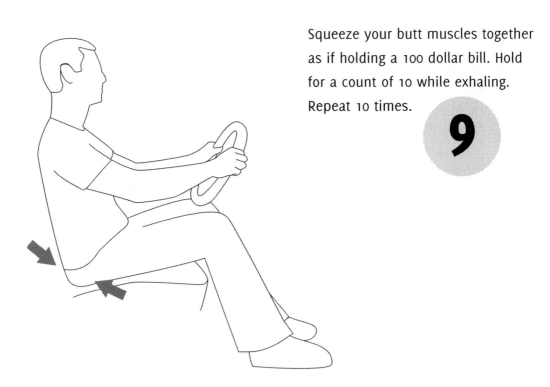

Turn slightly to your left. Place both hands
on the left side of the steering wheel at
9 and 10 O'clock. Try to pull the wheel
towards your right knee. Hold for a count of
10 while exhaling. Switch hands to right side
of wheel 2 and 3 O'clock. Repeat exercise.
Do each side twice.

10

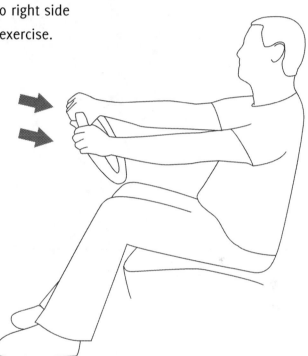

CHAPTER 8

FITNESS IN FLIGHT

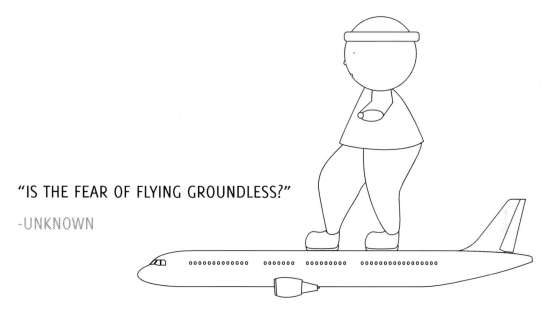

"IS THE FEAR OF FLYING GROUNDLESS?"

-UNKNOWN

TOP TEN WAYS AIRLINES ARE CUTTING BACK

10. PILOTS HAVE TO PAY FOR THEIR INFLIGHT COCKTAILS.

9. TICKET AGENTS URGING TRAVELERS TO STAY HOME.

8. TO MAXIMIZE SPACE, SEATS NO LONGER RECLINE A LUXURIOUS INCH-AND-A-HALF.

7. OXYGEN MASK COMPARTMENTS REPLACED WITH VIDEO POKER SCREENS.

6. INSTEAD OF COMPLIMENTARY PILLOWS, WADDED-UP CLOTHING PULLED OUT OF CHECKED LUGGAGE.

5. DIFFERENCE BETWEEN FIRST CLASS AND COACH? A BITE-SIZE 3 MUSKETEERS BAR.

4. FROM NOW ON, PLANES WILL TAXI FROM ONE DESTINATION TO ANOTHER ON THE INTERSTATE.

3. I DON'T KNOW, BUT HOW HARD IS IT TO OPEN THE PEANUTS, AM I RIGHT PEOPLE?

2. IN CASE OF WATER LANDING, YOUR ONLY FLOTATION DEVICE IS THE FAT GUY IN 16F.

1. INFLIGHT "MOVIE" IS HOME VIDEO OF THE PILOT "GETTIN' IT ON".

-DAVID LETTERMAN SHOW, MARCH 29, 2005

Even before 9/11 flying was a pain. Now it is an outright physical and mental ordeal that can exhaust you before you're even in the air. I understand the reason behind all these extra steps we now have to take for national security, but it sure doesn't make it any more enjoyable.

I had one, um...what's the word I'm looking for? Exasperating? Yes that's it – an exasperating experience at an airport that shall remain nameless. OK, it was LAX. They upset me so much, by the time I got to my seat I felt like I had run one of my marathons.

My least favorite part is going through the XRay machine. Take off your shoes, belt, jacket, bracelets, take out your cellphone, computer, film. Good grief, by the time I do all this I cannot locate my boarding pass, have no idea where my purse is and I have so many bins I need a check list to find all my stuff. I actually have a metal toe joint and I figured the toe would trigger the beeping machine. There were no chairs to sit on to tie my shoe laces and the crowd behind me was upset at how slowly I was getting organized. As I shuffled to the gate with loose laces and piles of stuff in my arms, nearly tripping most of the way, my water bottle was confiscated at the X-Ray machine upsetting me greatly. I always travel with water. When I arrived at the gate none of the stores were open. How exasperating...nothing to drink in flight.

Aaarrrgh.

We've all had bad pre-flight experiences. And they may make us feel stressed out angry and more tense than we should. And they can also put our bodies in knots. But once on the plane you have the opportunity to relieve that stress.

"What" you say? "Relief? Have you seen those seats in coach? Torquemada couldn't have designed anything more barbaric." What? Torquemada? Oh, he led the Spanish Inquisition. Really into torture. Stay with me here.

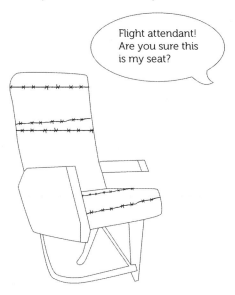

Flight attendant! Are you sure this is my seat?

Well, hang on a moment. Let's say you are taking a long flight somewhere. The airline recommends that you tap your toes, wiggle your fingers, turn your head, circle your ankles and generally move your parts during your flight so that the cabin attendant does not have to pry you out of your seat at the end of the flight, or worse you develop a clot and are DOA when the plane arrives. Gee, even the airline recommends wiggling those parts. Where have you heard that before?

With that in mind, here are some inflight tips.

First off, try for an aisle seat – they're the easiest to move your body parts around in. If you cannot get an aisle seat then try to sit next someone with a weak bladder, possibly someone older than you are. 😊 Every time they get up to use the restroom you get up too. Walk to the back of the plane or anywhere you can stretch, twist, bend, arch, march or anything else that will keep your bodily fluids moving around inflight.

(Quick Sidenote: Did you know there are seat belt extenders available for the plus size traveler? If you know this you are probably one of them. Were you also aware that on many flights to and from the Midwest or south the airlines are now running out of extenders? Hmmmm. Looks like we are in dire need of "parts-wiggling" in those areas of the country.)

OK, so now it's back those wonderful airline seats that no one fits in. Place a tote bag or book or jacket under one foot to unbalance the hip on that side. Continue to move the object from right to left foot during the entire flight. If you are lucky enough to get a pillow use it behind your back as a lumbar support. Both of these tips will help alleviate the back pain that so often accompanies long flights.

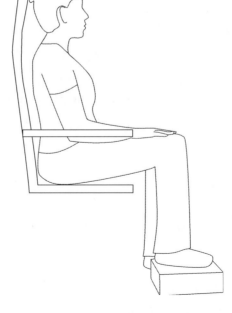

If that doesn't help, then you have to get up and move around. Here's some other activities you can do inflight:

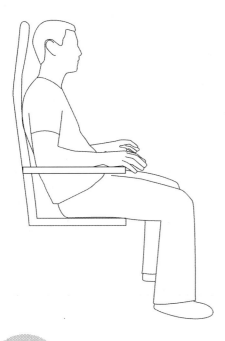

Place your elbows on the arm rests. Push down on the arm rests to lower your shoulders. This is like a chair push up. As you hold the position for a count of 10, breathe out and pull your navel in.

Hold your elbows at your waist and press into the seat behind you.

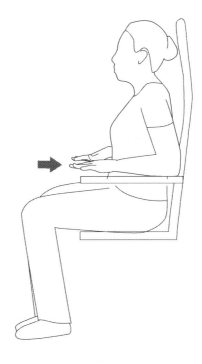

Pinch your midback (scapula) together but don't let your ribs open in front of your body.

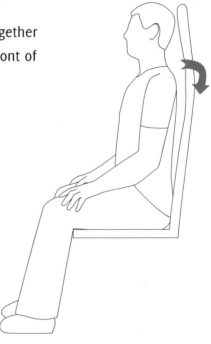

Place your right hand behind your head, side bend to your left for a great stretch. Alternate sides.

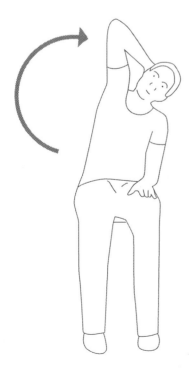

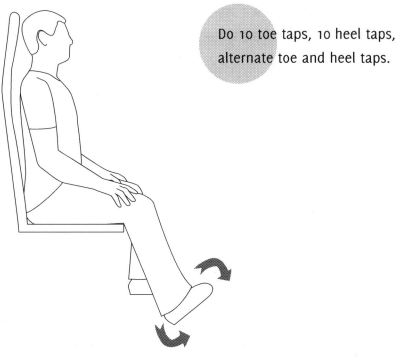

Do 10 toe taps, 10 heel taps, alternate toe and heel taps.

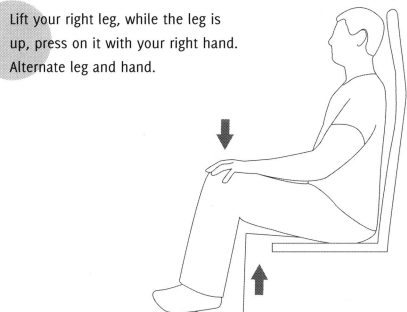

Lift your right leg, while the leg is up, press on it with your right hand. Alternate leg and hand.

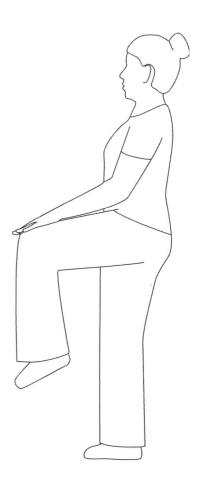

Do all the exercises standing when possible.

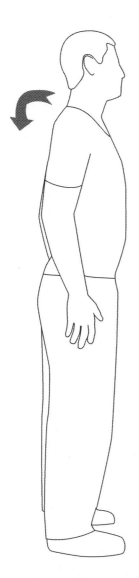

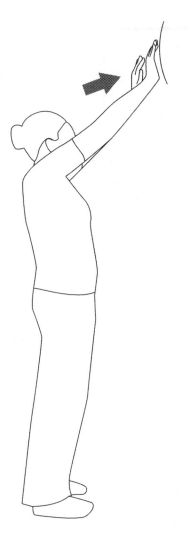

Reach both hands up toward the luggage bin. Press on the bin but don't open the bin. This exercise relaxes your neck and back.

CHAPTER 9

ARE YOU FIT ENOUGH FOR SEX?

"IT'S NOT HOW OLD YOU ARE, BUT HOW YOU ARE OLD."

—MARIE DRESSLER

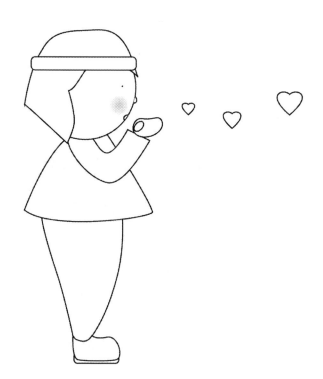
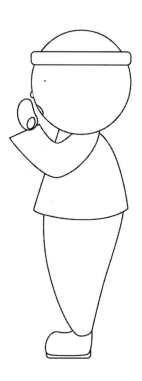

Let's get real here. With a certain population taking Vitamin V., there definitely is someone out there having sex. That being said, the question is, are you strong enough, fit enough and have enough endurance to do this? Sex takes energy. Do you have any energy? Sex takes endurance; can you walk up your staircase without panting? Sex takes strong glute muscles; do you sit on yours all day long so they have become spongy? Sex takes upper body strength, when was the last time you tried a push up? Okay, okay so you never looked at Sex this way before. There is a component of fitness in everything we do whether it is walking, working, playing etc. That means you need a fitness program even for Sex, so here it is.

VITAMIN V

QUADRUPED/FLYING TABLE POSITION

Get on all fours, which means on your knees and hands. Hands are under the shoulders, knees under the hips. First, find a neutral pelvis position with your head, mid back and tail in the same line if you were to put a yard stick on all three areas lengthwise. Let your stomach muscles go allowing your navel to pouch out. Then, without changing your back alignment gently pull in on your navel while breathing out. This exercise strengthens your mid back, wrists, shoulders, abs and pelvic floor. Do this exercise 10 times slowly.

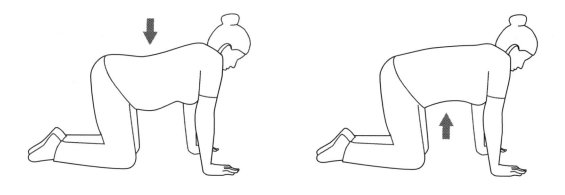

The next part of this exercise is more difficult. Slowly extend your right hand out in front of you and your left leg behind you. This is the Flying Table part of the position. Make sure you do not lean to one side. If you do lean start smaller by just extending your hand out in front of you. Return your hand to the floor then take your leg out and return it to the floor. When you can do each hand then leg do them both together. This provides balance, stability, strength and endurance.

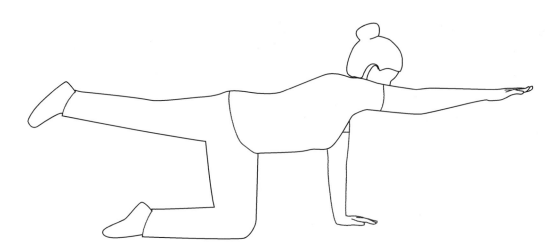

Once you have accomplished the flying table, tuck your toes under your feet and lift your knees a few inches off the floor. WOW! This works all your body parts. Do all these exercises 10 times and hold for a count of 10 while breathing out and pulling your ab muscles in.

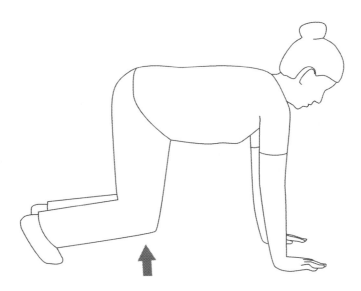

BRIDGING WITH FOOT PATTERNS

Lie on your back (supine) with your knees bent and feet flat on the floor, feet hip width apart. Let's focus on the glutes by doing several different positions for our bridges. Focus on squeezing the glutes to lift the buns off the ground to a plank position. That means not too high so there is no pain in your back or neck. Return your buns to the floor then squeeze the glutes again and lift them up to plank position. Do this exercise 10 times slowly using the glutes each time and not using your quads.

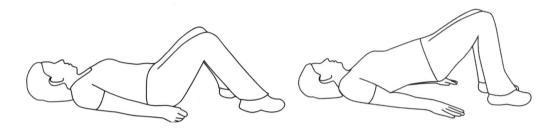

The second foot position is feet and knees together. Do the feet and knees together exercise 10 times slowly, squeezing the glutes each time you lift your buns off the floor.

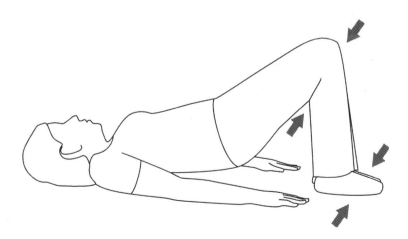

The third position is bottoms of the feet together with knees apart but not to wide apart. Once again squeeze the glutes to lift the buns off the floor. Do this exercise 10 times slowly.

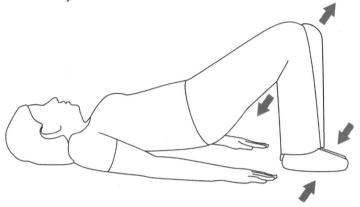

These next positions are more difficult and should not be tried until you master the previous positions.

The fourth position feet should be hip width apart as you bridge up using your glutes by squeezing them. Once you are in plank position, lift the right foot off the ground for a count of three, replace the foot then lift the left foot off the ground hold for a count of three and repeat this exercise 10 times on each leg. Once you get stronger hold the leg in the air longer like a count of 10. Then repeat on the other leg. The key to doing this exercise correctly is to not let your

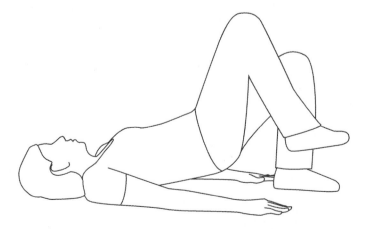

buns fall to the floor or that an arch is created in your back. Both suggest that you are no longer squeezing your buns and you are doing the exercise from your back muscles.

The fifth and final position when you are in a bridge is holding your opposing leg up toward the ceiling as you bring your buns to the floor and back up to bridge position. Do this exercise 10 times on each leg.

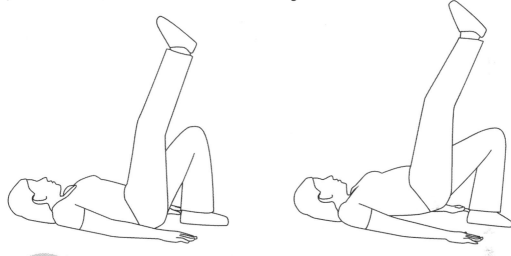

STAIR CLIMBING

Climbing stairs slowly is a great way to elevate your heart-rate to provide the endurance phase of your fitness program for Sex. Stair climbing is just plain a great exercise in general because it works your legs, breathing and pelvic floor. Have you seen all those machines at the gym that simulate stair climbing? Make sure you have consulted your medical care practitioner before doing this exercise. Be sure to begin slowly because you don't want to get dizzy on your way up or down the staircase. Hold on to the hand rail both directions up and down until you get used to doing this exercise. When you are proficient and confident then try to go up and down not using the hand rail. Each person will have a different degree of fitness so only do what is comfortable to you. If you are out of breath on the first one that will be all you do until one becomes easy. Then do two climbs. Add on the climbs only when the previous one becomes easy. If nothing else, if the elevator goes out in your building you will be the only one strong enough to take the stairs.

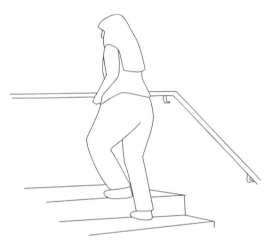

PELVIC FLOOR EXERCISE

When you are sitting at a red light in your car or when you are sitting in the movies before the lights go down or if you are watching a commercial between parts of your favorite TV show, PRETEND you are stopping your urine flow as if you were in the bathroom. This is called a KEGEL named for the doctor who invented it. Your pelvic floor is a group of muscles that hold your stuff in. Males and females have similar pelvic floor muscles. There is a slight difference because of the width of the female pelvis and organ differences but the muscles can be worked in the same manner. These muscles need to be worked like all muscles in your body. So, do this exercise five times and when you get stronger do this exercise 10 times.

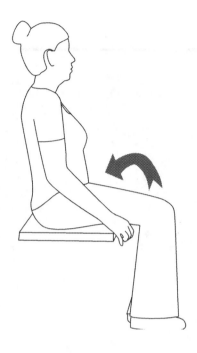

The featured exercises in this chapter work your muscles from the inside of your body to the outside of your body. The exercises help you get a stronger support system so you can garden without getting injured, carry heavy objects like your golf bag without getting injured, go for a walk with your grandchildren without getting injured and have sex – without getting injured.

CHAPTER 10

NOW THAT I'M PERFECT WHAT'S NEXT?

"ADVENTURE IS WORTHWHILE IN ITSELF."

-AMELIA EARHART

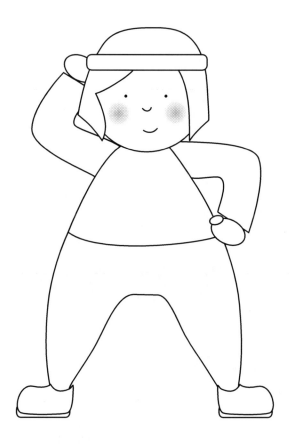

Getting to this point was exciting and hopefully you're a little motivated to go out and get moving. But this is a journey that never ends. There's no finish line. You will always be a work in progress. Growing old is not for sissies (that's good!). It is crucial to keep up your exercise and not throw it by the wayside. Maybe you can influence someone else – a family member – a friend – whoever to make a really positive change in their lives. That's huge. And then maybe that person can help someone else and so on and so on. You've started a chain!

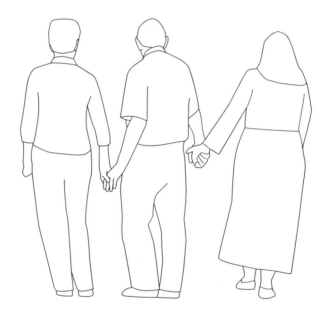

HERE ARE SOME TIPS TO HELP YOU STAY MOTIVATED AND KEEP WORKING:

Set Goals

Set goals for each week. Maybe working out three times this week, four days this week, or incorporating some type of aerobic or cardiovascular exercise for a particular week is a good beginning. Ten minutes more of aerobics, maybe, or trying to lose a pound in a week. Start the goals small and then build on them.

Keep a Diary

I've been keeping running diaries for 26 years. And I go back and look at those and find when I was able to accomplish a goal and how I felt. That's the exciting thing small goals that were obtainable. Look at your diary and see if you are hitting your goals.

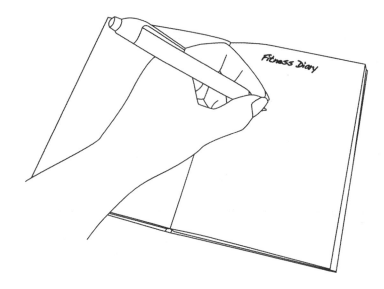

Get a Friend to Work with You

Misery loves company! If you are going to put yourself through this coming out or new you situation I'm sure you would love at least one of your friends to "enjoy" this journey with you. Find one of your "perky" friends to be your chief motivator. Someone who looks at the world through rosey glasses. You know the type, the glass is half full not half empty friend. Oh come on you must know at least one person who is still like that. Go look through your phone book of friends or your Blackberry. Have great faith that someone is still like that in this world. If you can find a friend like that, maybe they have a friend like that also. Get a few of these perky people together; they are the ones wearing *Life is Good* hats and shirts. Do whatever is necessary to keep you motivated.

Yay for You Point System

Set up a point system for doing basic life tasks and give yourself a Yay for You! for each task you do. For each task you do, add up the points each day and at the end of the week. Then try to earn more points each week and keep a log. Create a reward system of treats or something special just for you if you earn so many points.

Here are examples of **Yay for You** tasks and point list. Feel free to alter it based on your lifestyle:

ACTIVITIES TO DO AT HOME	POINTS EARNED	YAY FOR YOU!
Get out of bed and get dressed.	1	
While brushing your teeth, stand on one leg for a count of 30, repeat on other leg.	2 per leg	
If you have steps, walk down and up the steps 3 times.	3	
Go to the front door and push on the door with your right hand. Hold for a count of 10, switch hands and repeat.	2 per hand	
Pull on the door handle with the right hand. Hold for a count of 10, switch hands and repeat.	2 per hand	
Sit in a sturdy chair and get up from the chair 5 times.	3	

Continue sitting in the chair, tap your toes 40 times.	3	
Continue sitting in the chair, march one leg up and switch legs.	5	
Take your arms out from your sides and hold them there. Do 20 arm circles out ward and 20 arm circles inward. Repeat	5	
Get back in bed and roll onto your right side. Push yourself up to a sitting position on the right side 5 times. Switch and repeat on the other side.	5	
While on your bed, get on all fours or quadruped position. Lift one hand off the bed and balance. Replace hand back on the bed and lift other hand off the bed. Do 10 on each side.	5	
Sit on the side of the bed and place hands with straight arms behind you on the bed. Press down on the bed lifting your chest to the ceiling. This exercise is called a seated push-up. Do this 10 times.	5	
AT THE GROCERY STORE		
Park your car at the furthest parking space from the front entrance and walk.	3	
Take a cart and walk the perimeter of the store several times before going down the center aisles.	3	

Leave the cart on one aisle. Walk over to another aisle and choose products that you need to buy. Take turns carrying each item back to the cart.	1 per item	
Whenever you stop to read a label on a product stand on one leg and try to balance. Do this for each product you pick up.	1 per item	
At the check out stand, place items in cotton bags and carry them to your car.	5	
AT THE MOVIES		
Park your car at the furthest parking space from the front entrance and walk.	3	
Walk the escalator.	2	
Arrive early and buy your ticket so you can walk around the mall for at least 15 minutes.	3	
After the movie, walk the mall for another 15 minutes.	3	

If you do every exercise once, you can earn 70+ points which is very doable over several days. Read over the exercises and decide how many you will try on day one. Each day set a goal and try to achieve the goal. Once you are good at goal setting and achievements, then try to set higher goals like achieve more points each day. By the end of each week your points should be mounting higher.

Congratulations! Revel in your success of having completed all the work in this book. Realize that your real success is the journey you have taken and the self empowerment you have experienced. My friend JOY taught me to "get my mind right." That phrase helped me to stay on track, focus, keep a positive attitude and put one foot in front of the other. Every day when you awaken "get your mind right," suit up and show up and live life to the fullest. You earned the EXTENDED WARRANTY for your body parts; frame it and place it on your wall.

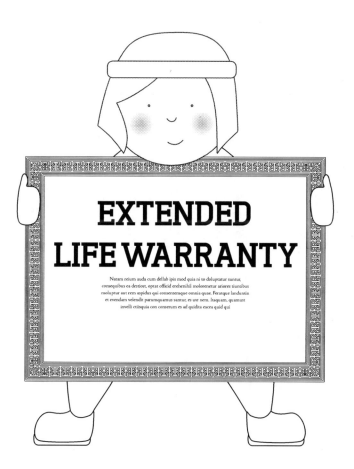